War On Drugs A Comprehensive Analysis

Arief Muinnudin

Published by Arief Muinnudin, 2024.

While every precaution has been taken in the preparation of this book, the publisher assumes no responsibility for errors or omissions, or for damages resulting from the use of the information contained herein.

WAR ON DRUGS A COMPREHENSIVE ANALYSIS

First edition. May 21, 2024.

Copyright © 2024 Arief Muinnudin.

ISBN: 979-8224625659

Written by Arief Muinnudin.

Table of Contents

War on Drugs: A Comprehensive Analysis

Chapter 1: Introduction to the War on Drugs

1.1 Definition and Scope

- Definition of the War on Drugs
- Scope and parameters
- Distinctions between drug use, abuse, and dependency

1.2 Historical Context

- Overview of drug use in ancient civilizations
- Evolution of drug policies over centuries
- Early 20th-century drug regulation efforts

1.3 Objectives and Goals

- Primary objectives of the War on Drugs
- Secondary and unintended goals
- Measures of success and failure

1.4 Methodology of the Book

- Multidisciplinary approach
- Sources and data collection
- Framework for analysis

1.5 Significance and Implications

- Societal impact
- Economic implications
- Global perspective

Chapter 2: The Early History of Drug Use and Regulation

2.1 Ancient Drug Use and Trade

- Drug use in Mesopotamia, Egypt, and China
- Role of drugs in religious and cultural practices
- Early trade routes and the spread of psychoactive substances

2.2 Opium Wars and International Trade

- Causes and consequences of the Opium Wars
- Impact on Sino-British relations
- Influence on global drug policies

2.3 Early Drug Regulation Policies

- The role of colonial powers in drug regulation
- The Hague Convention of 1912
- Domestic regulations in Europe and the Americas

2.4 The Birth of Modern Drug Laws

- The League of Nations and drug control
- The impact of World War II on drug policies
- Formation of the United Nations and the Single Convention on Narcotic Drugs (1961)

Chapter 3: The 20th Century and the Birth of the War on Drugs

3.1 The Harrison Narcotics Tax Act (1914)

- Legislative background
- Implementation and enforcement
- Societal and economic impacts

3.2 Prohibition Era and Alcohol

- The Volstead Act and the 18th Amendment
- Law enforcement challenges
- Lessons learned from alcohol prohibition

3.3 The Controlled Substances Act (1970)

- Legislative history and rationale
- Drug scheduling system
- Impact on drug policy and law enforcement

3.4 Richard Nixon and the Declaration of the War on Drugs

- Nixon's political strategy and rhetoric
- Key policies and initiatives
- Long-term implications of Nixon's declaration

3.5 Expansion under Subsequent Administrations

- Reagan's escalation and the Just Say No campaign
- The 1994 Crime Bill under Clinton
- Bush and Obama era policies

Chapter 4: The Role of Law Enforcement and the Criminal Justice System

4.1 Federal Agencies and Their Roles (DEA, FBI, etc.)

- History and evolution of the DEA
- Roles of the FBI and other federal agencies
- Coordination and conflicts between agencies

4.2 Mandatory Minimum Sentences

- Origins and rationale
- Impact on sentencing and incarceration rates
- Criticisms and calls for reform

4.3 Impact on Policing and Community Relations

- Community policing vs. aggressive drug enforcement
- Racial profiling and stop-and-frisk policies
- Case studies of police-community interactions

4.4 The Prison-Industrial Complex

- Growth of private prisons
- Economic incentives and political lobbying

4.5 Civil Asset Forfeiture

- Legal framework and procedures
- Financial impact on law enforcement agencies
- Controversies and abuses
- Reform efforts and legislative changes

4.6 Specialized Drug Courts and Diversion Programs

- History and development of drug courts
- Effectiveness and outcomes
- Comparison with traditional criminal justice approaches
- Examples of successful programs

4.7 The Role of Informants and Undercover Operations

- Use of confidential informants
- Legal and ethical considerations
- Impact on communities and trust in law enforcement

4.8 Surveillance and Privacy Issues

- Technological advancements in surveillance
- Legal battles over privacy and civil liberties
- Case studies of surveillance operations

4.9 International Law Enforcement Cooperation

- Role of INTERPOL and other international agencies
- Joint operations and task forces
- Challenges and successes in international cooperation

Chapter 5: Social and Cultural Impact of the War on Drugs

5.1 Media Representation and Public Perception

- Media portrayal of drug use and drug users
- Influence of movies, TV shows, and news coverage
- Role of public service announcements and anti-drug campaigns

5.2 The Crack Epidemic of the 1980s

- Origins and spread of crack cocaine
- Government and community responses
- Long-term impacts on affected communities

5.3 Hip-Hop Culture and Anti-Drug Messaging

- Evolution of drug-related themes in hip-hop
- Influence of prominent artists and lyrics
- Contrasting messages within the genre

5.4 The Stigma of Drug Addiction

- Societal attitudes towards addiction and addicts
- Impact on access to treatment and support services
- Efforts to reduce stigma and promote understanding

5.5 Drug Use in Subcultures and Marginalized Communities

- Drug use patterns among LGBTQ+ communities
- Impact on homeless populations
- Drug trends in rural vs. urban areas

5.6 Family Dynamics and the War on Drugs

- Impact of parental addiction on children
- Intergenerational cycles of drug abuse
- Support systems and community resources

5.7 Education and Youth Engagement

- School-based anti-drug programs (e.g., D.A.R.E.)
- Effectiveness of youth outreach initiatives
- Role of peer influence and social media

5.8 The Role of Religion and Faith-Based Organizations

- Religious perspectives on drug use and addiction
- Involvement of faith-based organizations in treatment and prevention
- Case studies of successful faith-based initiatives

Chapter 6: Economic Impact of the War on Drugs

6.1 Costs to Taxpayers

- Breakdown of federal, state, and local expenditures
- Long-term financial burden of drug enforcement and

incarceration
- Comparative analysis of prevention vs. enforcement costs

6.2 The Drug Trade and the Economy

- Economic scale of the global drug trade
- Impact on legitimate economies and businesses
- Money laundering and financial crime

6.3 Impact on Communities and Families

- Economic hardships faced by families of incarcerated individuals
- Loss of productivity and income in communities
- Effects on housing, education, and social services

6.4 Financial Incentives for Law Enforcement

- Analysis of asset forfeiture programs
- Grants and funding for drug enforcement initiatives
- Controversies over financial motivations

6.5 The Cost of Drug Treatment and Rehabilitation

- Funding and resource allocation for treatment programs
- Economic benefits of successful rehabilitation
- Comparison of treatment costs vs. incarceration costs

6.6 The Role of Pharmaceutical Companies

- Influence of the pharmaceutical industry on drug policy
- The opioid crisis and its economic impact
- Legal and financial consequences for pharmaceutical companies

6.7 Employment and the Labor Market

- Impact of drug convictions on employability
- Programs for reintegration and employment of former addicts
- Economic benefits of reducing drug-related unemployment

6.8 The Economics of Legalization and Decriminalization

- Financial outcomes of marijuana legalization
- Potential economic benefits of broader drug policy reform
- Case studies from states and countries with reformed drug policies

---

Chapter 7: International Dimensions of the War on Drugs

7.1 Drug Production and Trafficking Networks

- Overview of major drug-producing regions
- Key trafficking routes and methods
- Impact of globalization on drug trade dynamics

7.2 US Foreign Policy and Drug Eradication Programs

- Historical overview of US drug eradication efforts
- Analysis of programs like Plan Colombia
- Successes and failures of eradication strategies

7.3 The Role of Cartels and Organized Crime

- Structure and operations of major drug cartels
- Impact of cartel violence on societies
- Efforts to dismantle organized crime networks

7.4 Case Study: Colombia

- Historical context of Colombia's drug trade
- Government and US interventions
- Current challenges and future prospects

7.5 Case Study: Mexico

- Evolution of Mexico's drug cartels
- Impact of the Mérida Initiative
- Social and political consequences of the drug war

7.6 Case Study: Afghanistan

- Opium production and the Taliban
- International efforts to curb opium trade
- Impact on Afghan society and economy

7.7 Drug Policy in Europe

- Comparative analysis of drug policies in European countries
- Successes and challenges of harm reduction approaches
- Case studies from Portugal, Netherlands, and Switzerland

7.8 The Role of International Organizations

- United Nations Office on Drugs and Crime (UNODC)
- World Health Organization (WHO) and drug policy
- Collaboration and conflict between international bodies

7.9 Human Rights and International Drug Policy

- Impact of drug policies on human rights
- Efforts to align drug policy with human rights principles
- Case studies of human rights abuses linked to drug enforcement

Chapter 8: Health Implications and Drug Treatment

8.1 Addiction as a Disease

- Medical understanding of addiction
- Neuroscience of addiction
- Societal and policy implications of treating addiction as a disease

8.2 Public Health Approaches to Drug Use

- Principles of public health in drug policy
- Comparison of public health vs. criminal justice approaches
- Case studies of successful public health initiatives

8.3 Successes and Failures of Treatment Programs

- Evaluation of various treatment modalities (e.g., inpatient, outpatient, medication-assisted treatment)
- Factors contributing to successful treatment outcomes
- Challenges and barriers to effective treatment

8.4 The Rise of Harm Reduction Strategies

- Overview of harm reduction principles and practices
- Successes of needle exchange programs, supervised injection sites, and naloxone distribution
- Criticisms and controversies surrounding harm reduction

8.5 Mental Health and Co-occurring Disorders

- Intersection of addiction and mental health
- Approaches to integrated treatment
- Policy implications of dual diagnosis treatment

8.6 Access to Treatment and Healthcare Disparities

- Barriers to accessing treatment for marginalized populations
- Impact of healthcare systems and insurance policies
- Efforts to improve access and equity in treatment services

8.7 The Role of Non-Governmental Organizations (NGOs)

- Contributions of NGOs to drug treatment and harm reduction
- Case studies of successful NGO-led initiatives
- Challenges faced by NGOs in the drug policy landscape

8.8 Innovations in Addiction Treatment

- Emerging therapies and technologies
- Role of telehealth and digital tools in addiction treatment
- Future directions in addiction medicine

Chapter 9: Civil Rights and Legal Challenges

9.1 Racial Disparities in Drug Enforcement

- Historical context of racial disparities in drug laws
- Statistical analysis of disparities in arrests, convictions, and sentencing
- Impact on communities of color

9.2 Landmark Supreme Court Cases

- Key Supreme Court rulings impacting drug policy (e.g., Terry v. Ohio, Michigan v. Sitz)
- Analysis of judicial reasoning and legal precedents
- Long-term impact of these decisions on drug policy

9.3 The Impact on Civil Liberties

- Erosion of privacy rights and due process
- Impact of surveillance and data collection on civil liberties
- Balancing security and liberty in the context of drug enforcement

9.4 Advocacy and Legal Reforms

- Role of advocacy groups in promoting drug policy reform
- Major legal reforms and their impact
- Case studies of successful advocacy campaigns

9.5 Police Accountability and Reform

- Efforts to improve police accountability in drug enforcement
- Analysis of body camera programs, civilian oversight boards, and other reforms
- Case studies of police reform initiatives

9.6 Sentencing Reform and Alternatives to Incarceration

- Analysis of sentencing reform efforts (e.g., the Fair Sentencing Act)
- Role of diversion programs, restorative justice, and other alternatives
- Impact of sentencing reform on incarceration rates and recidivism

9.7 Juvenile Justice and Drug Policy

- Impact of drug policies on juvenile justice
- Treatment and rehabilitation programs for youth
- Efforts to reform juvenile drug laws

9.8 International Human Rights and Drug Policy

- Analysis of international human rights frameworks
- Efforts to align national drug policies with human rights standards
- Case studies of human rights violations linked to drug enforcement

---

Chapter 10: The Evolution of Drug Policy and Reform Movements

10.1 Decriminalization and Legalization Efforts

- Overview of global decriminalization and legalization trends
- Analysis of outcomes in countries/states that have decriminalized or legalized certain drugs
- Arguments for and against these approaches

10.2 The Medical Marijuana Movement

- History and development of the medical marijuana movement
- Scientific evidence and medical applications of cannabis
- Policy changes and their impact on public health and the economy

10.3 Changing Public Attitudes Towards Drugs

- Factors contributing to changing public attitudes
- Role of media, education, and personal experiences
- Impact of shifting attitudes on policy and enforcement

10.4 Policy Innovations and Alternatives

- Analysis of innovative drug policies (e.g., Portugal's

decriminalization model, Canada's safe supply programs)
- Evaluation of outcomes and lessons learned
- Potential for adaptation and implementation in other contexts

10.5 The Role of Technology in Drug Policy Reform

- Impact of technology on drug use and enforcement
- Use of data analytics, predictive policing, and digital tools in drug policy
- Future technological trends and their potential impact

10.6 Grassroots Movements and Community-Led Initiatives

- Role of grassroots movements in driving policy change
- Case studies of successful community-led initiatives
- Challenges and opportunities for grassroots activism

10.7 Legislative Efforts and Political Challenges

- Analysis of recent legislative efforts to reform drug policy
- Political dynamics and challenges in passing drug policy reforms
- Case studies of successful and unsuccessful legislative campaigns

10.8 International Perspectives on Drug Policy Reform

- Comparative analysis of drug policy reforms in different countries
- Role of international organizations and treaties in shaping national policies
- Future directions for global drug policy reform

Chapter 11: Case Studies and Personal Stories

11.1 Individual Stories of Addiction and Recovery

- Detailed personal narratives of addiction and recovery
- Impact of drug policies on individual lives
- Lessons learned from personal experiences

11.2 Impact on Families and Communities

- Case studies of families affected by drug addiction and enforcement
- Community responses and support networks
- Long-term effects on family dynamics and community cohesion

11.3 Success Stories of Drug Policy Reform

- Profiles of individuals and organizations that have successfully reformed drug policies
- Analysis of key factors contributing to their success
- Lessons learned and implications for future reforms

11.4 Interviews with Experts and Activists

- In-depth interviews with leading experts, activists, and policymakers
- Insights into the challenges and opportunities in drug policy reform
- Perspectives on the future of the War on Drugs

11.5 Case Study: Portugal's Decriminalization Model

- Detailed analysis of Portugal's drug decriminalization policy
- Outcomes and impact on public health and safety

- Lessons learned and potential for replication in other contexts

11.6 Case Study: Colorado and Marijuana Legalization

- History and development of marijuana legalization in Colorado
- Economic, social, and public health impacts
- Analysis of regulatory challenges and successes

11.7 Case Study: The Philippines and Duterte's Drug War

- Overview of President Duterte's aggressive anti-drug campaign
- Human rights violations and international response
- Impact on Filipino society and potential for policy change

11.8 The Role of Social Movements and Advocacy

- Analysis of social movements advocating for drug policy reform
- Role of advocacy organizations and community groups
- Case studies of successful advocacy efforts

Chapter 12: The Future of the War on Drugs

12.1 Emerging Drug Trends and Threats

- Analysis of new and emerging drugs (e.g., synthetic opioids, designer drugs)
- Impact of changing drug use patterns on policy and enforcement
- Strategies for addressing emerging drug threats

12.2 Technological Innovations in Drug Enforcement

- Overview of technological advancements in drug enforcement
- Potential benefits and risks of new technologies
- Future trends and their implications for drug policy

12.3 Global Perspectives on Drug Policy

- Comparative analysis of drug policies around the world
- Impact of globalization on drug enforcement and policy
- Role of international cooperation in shaping future drug policies

12.4 Vision for a Post-Prohibition World

- Analysis of the potential for a post-prohibition approach to drug policy
- Economic, social, and public health implications of ending prohibition
- Roadmap for transitioning to a post-prohibition world

12.5 Policy Innovations and Best Practices

- Overview of innovative policy approaches and best practices
- Case studies of successful policy innovations
- Recommendations for implementing best practices in different contexts

12.6 Future Directions for Drug Treatment and Harm Reduction

- Emerging trends in addiction treatment and harm reduction
- Role of new therapies and technologies
- Policy implications of advances in treatment and harm reduction

12.7 The Role of Education and Public Awareness

- Importance of education and public awareness in shaping drug policy
- Strategies for effective public education campaigns
- Case studies of successful education and awareness initiatives

12.8 Building a More Just and Effective Drug Policy

- Key principles for a more just and effective drug policy
- Role of stakeholders in driving policy change
- Vision for the future of drug policy and the War on Drugs

Chapter 13: Conclusion and Recommendations

13.1 Summary of Key Findings

- Recap of the major findings from each chapter
- Synthesis of key insights and conclusions

13.2 Policy Recommendations

- Detailed policy recommendations based on the analysis presented in the book
- Specific actions for policymakers, practitioners, and advocates

13.3 The Path Forward

- Steps needed to move towards a more effective and just approach to drug policy
- Role of various stakeholders in driving change

13.4 Final Reflections

- Reflections on the lessons learned from the War on Drugs
- Hope for a better future and the potential for meaningful change

13.5 Call to Action

- Encouragement for readers to get involved in drug policy reform
- Resources and organizations to support for those interested in advocacy

Chapter 1: Introduction to the War on Drugs

1.1 Definition and Scope

The "War on Drugs" is a term coined to describe the United States government's campaign of prohibition, military aid, and military intervention aimed at reducing the illegal drug trade. The campaign was initiated by President Richard Nixon in June 1971, declaring drug abuse as "public enemy number one." The term has since evolved to encompass a range of government policies designed to curb the production, distribution, and consumption of illicit substances.

The scope of the War on Drugs is vast, encompassing a variety of strategies including criminal justice measures, public health initiatives, and international cooperation. It targets both the supply and demand sides of the drug equation, addressing production, trafficking, and consumption. This multi-faceted approach aims to disrupt drug markets, incarcerate offenders, and reduce drug use through prevention and treatment programs.

1.2 Historical Context

Drug use has been a part of human history for millennia, with evidence of psychoactive substance use dating back to ancient civilizations. The Sumerians used opium, the Chinese consumed tea and later opium, and indigenous cultures in the Americas used coca leaves and peyote. Drug use was often tied to religious rituals, medical practices, and social activities.

In the 19th century, drugs like opium, morphine, and cocaine were widely used and largely unregulated. The widespread availability of these substances led to various social problems, prompting the first regulatory measures. The Pure Food and Drug Act of 1906 marked one of the earliest attempts to control drug use by requiring accurate labeling of ingredients in medications.

The early 20th century saw a more aggressive stance with the Harrison Narcotics Tax Act of 1914, which regulated and taxed the production and distribution of opiates and coca products. This act laid the groundwork for future drug prohibition policies and established a legal framework that would evolve into the modern War on Drugs.

1.3 Objectives and Goals

The primary objective of the War on Drugs is to reduce the availability and consumption of illicit drugs. This goal is pursued through various means, including law enforcement, border control, international cooperation, and public education campaigns. The overarching aim is to protect public health and safety by curbing drug-related crime and addiction.

Secondary goals include dismantling drug trafficking organizations, reducing drug-related violence, and mitigating the social and economic impacts of drug abuse. These objectives are often pursued through stringent law enforcement measures, including mandatory minimum sentencing, increased policing, and military interventions in drug-producing regions.

Despite its clear objectives, the War on Drugs has faced criticism for its perceived failure to achieve long-term reductions in drug use and its disproportionate impact on marginalized communities. Measuring success has been challenging, as indicators like drug availability and usage rates have shown mixed results over the decades.

1.4 Methodology of the Book

This book adopts a multidisciplinary approach to examine the War on Drugs, drawing on historical analysis, sociological research, economic studies, and public health perspectives. Primary sources include government documents, legal texts, and interviews with policymakers, law enforcement officials, and individuals affected by drug policies. Secondary sources include academic research, news articles, and reports from non-governmental organizations.

Data collection involves both quantitative and qualitative methods, analyzing statistics on drug use, incarceration rates, economic costs, and public health outcomes. Case studies from different countries and communities provide a detailed look at the varied impacts of drug policies.

The analytical framework integrates theories from criminology, public policy, and health sciences to evaluate the effectiveness and consequences of the War on Drugs. This comprehensive approach aims to provide a balanced and nuanced understanding of the issue.

1.5 Significance and Implications

The War on Drugs has had profound implications for society, economy, and global politics. It has reshaped criminal justice systems, influenced international relations, and affected millions of lives worldwide. The social significance is evident in the widespread stigma attached to drug users, the racial disparities in drug enforcement, and the community disruptions caused by mass incarceration.

Economically, the War on Drugs has resulted in substantial public expenditure on law enforcement, prisons, and drug treatment programs. The illicit drug trade, meanwhile, remains a significant component of the global economy, with vast sums of money flowing through criminal networks and affecting legitimate markets.

On a global scale, the War on Drugs has shaped diplomatic relations, with countries like the United States exerting pressure on drug-producing nations to adopt stricter control measures. International drug control treaties and cooperative efforts reflect the interconnected nature of the problem and the shared responsibility for addressing it.

Understanding the War on Drugs is crucial for policymakers, researchers, and the public as it provides insights into the complexities of drug control, the effectiveness of various strategies, and the unintended consequences of prohibitionist policies. This book aims to contribute to this understanding by offering a thorough analysis of the historical, social, economic, and political dimensions of the War on Drugs.

Chapter 2: The Early History of Drug Use and Regulation

2.1 Ancient Drug Use and Trade

The use of psychoactive substances is as old as human civilization itself. Archaeological evidence indicates that ancient cultures across the globe used various natural substances for medicinal, religious, and recreational purposes. In Mesopotamia, the Sumerians referred to the opium poppy as the "joy plant" around 3400 BCE. The Egyptians used opium in religious ceremonies and as a remedy for ailments.

China has a long history of drug use, with tea being consumed for its stimulating effects as early as 2737 BCE. The use of opium became prevalent by the 7th century, eventually leading to significant social and economic impacts. In the Americas, indigenous peoples used coca leaves and peyote in their traditional practices, often in spiritual contexts.

The trade of these substances facilitated cultural exchanges and economic relationships between ancient civilizations. Opium, for example, was traded along the Silk Road, connecting the East and West and influencing medical practices across continents.

2.2 Opium Wars and International Trade

The Opium Wars in the mid-19th century marked a significant turning point in the global drug trade and international relations. The First Opium War (1839-1842) and the Second Opium War (1856-1860) were conflicts between China and Britain, primarily over the British trade of opium in China.

The British East India Company had established a profitable trade network, exporting opium from India to China in exchange for tea and other goods. The widespread addiction in China led to social and economic problems, prompting the Qing Dynasty to take measures to curb opium imports.

British resistance to these measures resulted in military conflict, ultimately leading to China's defeat and the imposition of the Treaty of Nanking and the Treaty of Tientsin. These treaties forced China to cede territory, pay reparations, and allow the continued importation of opium, significantly impacting Chinese sovereignty and setting the stage for future foreign interventions.

2.3 Early Drug Regulation Policies

The 19th and early 20th centuries saw the beginnings of formal drug regulation. The growing recognition of the harms associated with uncontrolled drug use led to the establishment of national and international regulatory frameworks.

In the United States, the Pure Food and Drug Act of 1906 required accurate labeling of ingredients in medications, marking a significant step towards consumer protection. The Harrison Narcotics Tax Act of 1914 further regulated opiates and coca products, introducing a tax system to control their distribution.

Internationally, The Hague Convention of 1912 was the first international treaty aimed at controlling the opium trade. It sought to limit the production, distribution, and consumption of opium and its derivatives, laying the groundwork for future international drug control efforts.

2.4 The Birth of Modern Drug Laws

The aftermath of World War I and the establishment of the League of Nations provided a new platform for international drug control. The

League's efforts culminated in the 1925 Opium Convention, which expanded the scope of drug control to include coca and cannabis.

The interwar period saw increasing national efforts to control drug use, influenced by both international treaties and domestic concerns. The United States continued to tighten its drug laws, culminating in the Marijuana Tax Act of 1937, which effectively criminalized cannabis.

The formation of the United Nations after World War II brought renewed focus on international drug control. The 1961 Single Convention on Narcotic Drugs consolidated previous treaties and aimed to limit the production and supply of narcotic drugs to medical and scientific purposes. This convention remains a cornerstone of the international drug control regime, reflecting a prohibitionist approach that has shaped global drug policies for decades.

2.5 The Role of Racism in Early Drug Laws

The development of early drug laws in the United States and other countries was often influenced by racial and ethnic prejudices. Anti-Chinese sentiment played a significant role in the enactment of laws targeting opium use in the late 19th and early 20th centuries. The Chinese Exclusion Act of 1882 and subsequent opium laws were partly a response to the perception that Chinese immigrants and their opium dens were corrupting American society.

Similarly, anti-Mexican sentiment influenced the criminalization of marijuana. During the early 20th century, Mexican immigrants were often associated with marijuana use. Media portrayals and political rhetoric framed marijuana as a dangerous drug used primarily by Mexican laborers, leading to the Marijuana Tax Act of 1937, which effectively banned the substance.

African Americans were also disproportionately targeted by early drug laws. The association of cocaine use with African Americans in the early 20th century fueled racist fears and led to harsher penalties for cocaine-related offenses. This pattern of racialized drug enforcement laid the foundation for future disparities in the War on Drugs.

2.6 The Emergence of Federal Agencies

The creation of federal agencies dedicated to drug control marked a significant shift in the enforcement and regulation of drug laws. In 1930, the Federal Bureau of Narcotics (FBN) was established within the Department of the Treasury, with Harry J. Anslinger as its first commissioner. Anslinger was a staunch advocate for strict drug prohibition and played a key role in shaping U.S. drug policy for over three decades.

Under Anslinger's leadership, the FBN aggressively pursued drug traffickers and users, often employing sensationalist propaganda to garner public support for its initiatives. The agency's efforts culminated in the passage of the Boggs Act in 1951 and the Narcotic Control Act in 1956, both of which imposed severe mandatory minimum sentences for drug offenses.

The FBN was later merged with other agencies to form the Bureau of Narcotics and Dangerous Drugs (BNDD) in 1968, which eventually became the Drug Enforcement Administration (DEA) in 1973. The DEA, as the primary federal agency responsible for enforcing drug laws, continues to play a central role in the War on Drugs.

2.7 International Drug Control Treaties

The mid-20th century saw the consolidation of international efforts to control drug trafficking and abuse. The United Nations took a leading role in coordinating global drug policy through a series of international treaties.

The 1961 Single Convention on Narcotic Drugs aimed to limit the production and supply of narcotic drugs to medical and scientific purposes, establishing a framework for international cooperation. The convention also created the International Narcotics Control Board (INCB) to monitor compliance and ensure the availability of controlled substances for legitimate uses.

Subsequent treaties, including the 1971 Convention on Psychotropic Substances and the 1988 United Nations Convention Against Illicit Traffic in Narcotic Drugs and Psychotropic Substances, expanded the scope of international drug control to include a wider range of substances and emphasized the importance of criminal justice measures in combating drug trafficking.

These treaties reflect a prohibitionist approach that has dominated global drug policy for decades, influencing national laws and enforcement practices around the world.

2.8 The Nixon Administration and the Declaration of the War on Drugs

The modern War on Drugs was formally declared by President Richard Nixon in June 1971. In a speech to Congress, Nixon identified drug abuse as "public enemy number one" and called for a comprehensive national strategy to combat it. This declaration marked a significant escalation in the federal government's commitment to addressing the drug problem.

The Nixon administration established the Special Action Office for Drug Abuse Prevention (SAODAP) to coordinate federal drug policy and launched the National Institute on Drug Abuse (NIDA) to support research on drug abuse and addiction. Nixon's approach included both supply-side measures, such as law enforcement and interdiction efforts, and demand-side measures, such as prevention and treatment programs.

Despite this balanced approach, the emphasis on law enforcement and punitive measures set the tone for future administrations. The Controlled Substances Act of 1970, which classified drugs into schedules based on their potential for abuse and medical use, provided a legal framework for the federal government's drug control efforts.

Chapter 3: Escalation of the War on Drugs in the 1980s

3.1 The Reagan Administration's Approach

The 1980s saw a significant escalation in the War on Drugs under President Ronald Reagan. Reagan's administration adopted a hardline stance on drug use and trafficking, prioritizing law enforcement and punitive measures over prevention and treatment.

The Anti-Drug Abuse Act of 1986, a cornerstone of Reagan's drug policy, introduced mandatory minimum sentences for drug offenses and increased funding for law enforcement and interdiction efforts. The act also created the Office of National Drug Control Policy (ONDCP) to coordinate federal drug policy and oversee anti-drug initiatives.

Reagan's rhetoric and policies contributed to a dramatic increase in drug-related arrests and incarcerations, disproportionately affecting minority communities. The administration's "Just Say No" campaign, led by First Lady Nancy Reagan, aimed to prevent drug use through public education and awareness, but its effectiveness was widely debated.

3.2 The Crack Cocaine Epidemic

The mid-1980s witnessed the emergence of crack cocaine, a potent and inexpensive form of cocaine that became widely available in urban areas. The crack epidemic had devastating social and economic impacts, particularly in African American communities.

The media played a significant role in shaping public perception of the crack epidemic, often portraying it as a crisis of unprecedented proportions. Sensationalist coverage contributed to widespread fear and panic, influencing public support for harsh anti-drug measures.

The Anti-Drug Abuse Act of 1986 included provisions that established a 100:1 sentencing disparity between crack and powder cocaine offenses, leading to disproportionately harsh penalties for crack users, who were predominantly African American. This disparity contributed to significant racial disparities in drug-related incarcerations, exacerbating existing social inequalities.

3.3 Mandatory Minimum Sentences and Mass Incarceration

The introduction of mandatory minimum sentences for drug offenses in the 1980s marked a significant shift in U.S. criminal justice policy. These laws required judges to impose fixed, severe sentences for specific drug offenses, limiting judicial discretion and leading to a dramatic increase in the prison population.

Mandatory minimums disproportionately affected low-level drug offenders and contributed to the phenomenon of mass incarceration. By the late 1980s and early 1990s, the U.S. prison population had skyrocketed, with a significant portion of inmates serving long sentences for non-violent drug offenses.

The social and economic costs of mass incarceration have been profound, affecting families, communities, and entire generations. The racial disparities in sentencing and incarceration have further entrenched systemic inequalities, prompting calls for reform and a reevaluation of punitive drug policies.

3.4 The Role of Media and Public Perception

The media has played a crucial role in shaping public perception of the drug problem and influencing drug policy. Throughout the 1980s, news coverage of the crack cocaine epidemic, drug-related violence, and high-profile arrests fueled public fear and supported the call for tougher drug laws.

Media portrayals often emphasized the dangers of drug use and the need for a strong law enforcement response, reinforcing the narrative of the War on Drugs. Public service announcements and anti-drug campaigns, such as the Partnership for a Drug-Free America's "This Is Your Brain on Drugs" campaign, aimed to educate the public and deter drug use through dramatic imagery and messaging.

The impact of media coverage on public perception and policy cannot be overstated. It has shaped the national conversation on drugs, influenced legislative action, and contributed to the stigmatization of drug users.

3.5 Community Impact and Response

The escalation of the War on Drugs in the 1980s had profound impacts on communities across the United States, particularly in urban areas with high levels of drug activity. The aggressive law enforcement tactics and punitive sentencing policies disproportionately affected African American and Latino communities, leading to widespread social and economic disruption.

Communities responded to the challenges posed by the drug epidemic and the War on Drugs in various ways. Grassroots organizations and community leaders mobilized to address the root causes of drug abuse, provide support for affected individuals and families, and advocate for policy changes.

Efforts to improve community-police relations, increase access to drug treatment and rehabilitation services, and promote economic development have been central to these community-based initiatives. The resilience and activism of affected communities have played a crucial role in shaping the ongoing debate over drug policy and reform.

Chapter 4: The War on Drugs and Public Health

4.1 Drug Abuse and Addiction as Public Health Issues

Drug abuse and addiction are complex public health issues that affect individuals, families, and communities. They are characterized by a compulsive need to seek and use drugs despite harmful consequences. The medical community increasingly views addiction as a chronic disease that alters brain function and behavior, requiring comprehensive treatment and long-term management.

Understanding addiction as a public health issue necessitates a shift from punitive approaches to strategies focused on prevention, treatment, and harm reduction. Addressing the root causes of addiction, such as trauma, mental health issues, and socio-economic factors, is crucial for effective intervention.

Public health approaches emphasize the importance of early intervention, access to healthcare, and supportive services to help individuals recover from addiction and reintegrate into society. This perspective contrasts sharply with the punitive measures traditionally associated with the War on Drugs.

4.2 The Impact of Criminalization on Health Outcomes

The criminalization of drug use has significant negative consequences for public health. Incarceration exposes individuals to health risks, including infectious diseases such as HIV and hepatitis, which can spread in crowded prison environments. The lack of adequate healthcare in prisons exacerbates these issues, leading to poor health outcomes for incarcerated individuals.

Criminalization also creates barriers to accessing healthcare and treatment services. Fear of legal repercussions can deter individuals from seeking help, and those with criminal records may face discrimination in healthcare settings. The stigma associated with drug use further marginalizes individuals, making it harder for them to receive the support they need.

The emphasis on punitive measures has diverted resources away from public health initiatives that could more effectively address the underlying causes of drug abuse and addiction. This misallocation of resources has hindered efforts to improve health outcomes and reduce the social and economic costs of drug addiction.

4.3 The Role of Treatment and Rehabilitation Programs

Effective treatment and rehabilitation programs are essential components of a public health approach to drug addiction. These programs offer a range of services, including medical detoxification, behavioral therapy, counseling, and support for co-occurring mental health disorders.

Evidence-based treatment approaches, such as medication-assisted treatment (MAT) for opioid addiction, have proven effective in helping individuals achieve and maintain recovery. MAT combines medications like methadone or buprenorphine with counseling and behavioral therapies to address the physical and psychological aspects of addiction.

Rehabilitation programs also focus on social reintegration, providing support for education, employment, and housing. This holistic approach recognizes that recovery is not just about abstaining from drugs but also about rebuilding a stable and fulfilling life.

Despite their effectiveness, access to treatment and rehabilitation programs remains limited, particularly for marginalized populations.

Expanding these services and integrating them into broader healthcare systems is crucial for addressing the public health crisis of drug addiction.

4.4 Harm Reduction Strategies

Harm reduction is a public health strategy aimed at minimizing the negative health, social, and legal impacts associated with drug use. It acknowledges that while abstinence may be the ideal outcome, it is not always feasible for everyone. Instead, harm reduction focuses on reducing the risks and harms of drug use.

Examples of harm reduction strategies include needle exchange programs, supervised injection sites, and the distribution of naloxone to prevent opioid overdoses. These interventions have been shown to reduce the spread of infectious diseases, prevent overdose deaths, and connect individuals with healthcare and treatment services.

Harm reduction approaches are often controversial because they challenge traditional abstinence-only models and punitive drug policies. However, a growing body of evidence supports their effectiveness in improving health outcomes and reducing the social harms associated with drug use.

4.5 Case Studies of Public Health Approaches

Several countries and regions have implemented public health approaches to drug policy with notable success. These case studies provide valuable lessons for other jurisdictions considering similar reforms.

Portugal's Decriminalization Model

Portugal's decision to decriminalize all drugs in 2001 marked a significant shift from punitive to public health-focused drug policy.

Under this model, drug possession for personal use is treated as an administrative offense rather than a criminal one. Individuals found with small amounts of drugs are referred to a "dissuasion commission" composed of healthcare professionals and social workers, who assess their needs and recommend treatment, counseling, or fines.

The results of Portugal's decriminalization have been positive. Drug-related deaths, HIV infection rates, and overall drug use have decreased, while access to treatment and harm reduction services has improved. Portugal's experience demonstrates the potential benefits of treating drug use as a health issue rather than a criminal one.

Switzerland's Heroin-Assisted Treatment

Switzerland's heroin-assisted treatment program, introduced in the 1990s, provides medically prescribed heroin to individuals with severe addiction who have not responded to other treatments. The program includes comprehensive healthcare, social services, and psychosocial support.

Studies have shown that heroin-assisted treatment reduces illicit drug use, criminal activity, and health problems while improving social reintegration and quality of life for participants. The success of this program has influenced drug policy in other countries and highlighted the importance of evidence-based interventions.

4.6 Barriers to Implementing Public Health Approaches

Despite the evidence supporting public health approaches to drug policy, several barriers hinder their widespread adoption. These include political resistance, social stigma, and the entrenched interests of those who benefit from the status quo of punitive measures.

Political resistance often stems from the perception that public health approaches are "soft on crime" and could lead to increased drug use.

This perception is fueled by sensationalist media coverage and public fear, making it challenging for policymakers to advocate for reform.

Social stigma against drug users perpetuates discriminatory attitudes and practices, both in society at large and within healthcare systems. This stigma can discourage individuals from seeking help and undermine the effectiveness of harm reduction and treatment programs.

Finally, the financial and institutional interests of law enforcement agencies, private prison operators, and other stakeholders in the criminal justice system can create significant obstacles to reform. Addressing these barriers requires concerted efforts to educate the public, build political will, and reallocate resources towards evidence-based public health strategies.

Chapter 5: The International Dimensions of the War on Drugs

5.1 The Global Drug Trade

The global drug trade is a complex and highly lucrative enterprise that spans multiple continents and involves a vast network of producers, traffickers, and consumers. It is driven by the high demand for illegal substances in consumer countries and the economic incentives for producers in drug-source countries.

Major drug-producing regions include Latin America, where cocaine and cannabis are produced; Southeast Asia's Golden Triangle, known for opium production; and Afghanistan, the world's largest producer of opium. These regions supply drugs to major consumer markets in North America, Europe, and Asia.

The illicit drug trade generates significant revenue for criminal organizations, fueling corruption, violence, and instability in producing and transit countries. Efforts to combat the drug trade involve complex international cooperation and coordination among law enforcement agencies, governments, and international organizations.

5.2 The Role of International Organizations

International organizations play a crucial role in coordinating global drug control efforts. The United Nations Office on Drugs and Crime (UNODC) is the primary body responsible for international drug policy, working to promote drug control treaties, provide technical assistance, and support capacity-building initiatives in member states.

The International Narcotics Control Board (INCB) monitors the implementation of international drug control treaties and ensures that countries comply with their obligations. The INCB also works to balance the need for controlled substances for medical and scientific purposes with efforts to prevent their diversion into illegal channels.

Other organizations, such as Interpol and the World Health Organization (WHO), also contribute to global drug control efforts by facilitating international cooperation, conducting research, and promoting public health approaches to drug policy.

5.3 U.S. Influence on Global Drug Policy

The United States has played a dominant role in shaping global drug policy, using its political and economic influence to promote prohibitionist approaches. U.S. drug policy has historically emphasized law enforcement, interdiction, and eradication efforts, often pressuring other countries to adopt similar measures.

U.S. foreign aid and military assistance are frequently tied to drug control efforts, with programs like Plan Colombia providing substantial support for drug eradication and interdiction in Latin America. While these efforts have had some success in reducing drug production and trafficking, they have also been criticized for exacerbating violence, human rights abuses, and social instability in affected regions.

The U.S. has also been instrumental in the development and enforcement of international drug control treaties, ensuring that prohibitionist principles are enshrined in global drug policy. This influence has shaped the approach of many countries, although recent shifts towards more progressive policies in some regions indicate a growing divergence from U.S. strategies.

5.4 Case Study: Plan Colombia

Plan Colombia, launched in 2000, is one of the most significant U.S.-funded drug control initiatives in Latin America. The plan aimed to reduce coca cultivation and cocaine production through a combination of military assistance, aerial fumigation, and alternative development programs.

While Plan Colombia achieved some success in reducing coca cultivation and disrupting drug trafficking organizations, it also had significant unintended consequences. Aerial fumigation caused environmental damage and displaced rural communities, contributing to social unrest and exacerbating the internal conflict in Colombia.

Critics argue that Plan Colombia's heavy emphasis on military solutions overlooked the underlying socio-economic factors driving the drug trade. Despite substantial U.S. investment, the program did not achieve a sustainable reduction in drug production, highlighting the limitations of prohibitionist approaches.

5.5 The Impact on Producer and Transit Countries

Producer and transit countries bear the brunt of the War on Drugs, facing significant social, economic, and political challenges as a result of their involvement in the global drug trade. These countries often experience high levels of violence, corruption, and instability, undermining development and governance.

In Latin America, countries like Mexico, Colombia, and Honduras have been particularly affected by drug-related violence and criminal activity. The presence of powerful drug cartels and the militarization of anti-drug efforts have led to widespread human rights abuses and social dislocation.

In Southeast Asia, the Golden Triangle region continues to grapple with the challenges of opium production and trafficking. Efforts to reduce drug cultivation through eradication and alternative development programs have had mixed results, often failing to provide sustainable livelihoods for affected communities.

Transit countries, such as those in West Africa, have emerged as key nodes in global drug trafficking routes. These countries face increasing pressure from international drug control efforts while struggling with limited resources and capacity to address the complex challenges posed by the drug trade.

5.6 Moving Towards International Drug Policy Reform

The growing recognition of the limitations and negative consequences of prohibitionist drug policies has sparked calls for international drug policy reform. Advocates argue for a shift towards approaches that prioritize public health, human rights, and sustainable development.

Recent years have seen a number of countries experimenting with alternative drug policies, such as decriminalization, legalization, and harm reduction strategies. These initiatives challenge the traditional prohibitionist framework and offer new models for addressing the global drug problem.

International drug policy reform requires a coordinated and collaborative effort among countries, international organizations, and civil society. It involves rethinking existing treaties, reallocating resources towards evidence-based interventions, and fostering a global dialogue that embraces diverse perspectives and experiences.

Chapter 6: The Social and Economic Costs of the War on Drugs

6.1 Economic Impact

The War on Drugs has significant economic implications, affecting government spending, law enforcement budgets, healthcare costs, and productivity. The allocation of resources towards drug control efforts, including policing, incarceration, and interdiction, represents a substantial financial burden on taxpayers.

Economic analyses have shown that the costs of enforcing drug prohibition often outweigh the benefits, with limited success in reducing drug availability or use. The high costs of incarceration, particularly for non-violent drug offenders, strain public budgets and divert funds from other critical social programs.

Moreover, the illicit drug trade generates significant revenue for criminal organizations, contributing to underground economies and undermining legitimate markets. The economic incentives for drug production and trafficking persist despite law enforcement efforts, highlighting the challenges of prohibitionist policies.

6.2 Social Costs

The social costs of the War on Drugs are profound, impacting individuals, families, and communities in myriad ways. Mass incarceration resulting from drug-related convictions has led to family disruption, community disintegration, and intergenerational cycles of poverty and incarceration.

The criminalization of drug use has also perpetuated stigma and discrimination against drug users, leading to social exclusion, limited employment opportunities, and barriers to accessing education and healthcare. This marginalization exacerbates existing inequalities and contributes to social unrest and disenfranchisement.

Furthermore, the War on Drugs has fueled violence and conflict, both domestically and internationally. Drug-related crime, including trafficking, turf wars, and gang violence, has claimed countless lives and destabilized communities. The militarization of drug control efforts has led to human rights abuses, extrajudicial killings, and erosion of civil liberties in affected regions.

6.3 Health Consequences

The health consequences of the War on Drugs extend beyond addiction and overdose to encompass a range of public health issues. Criminalization and stigma create barriers to accessing healthcare and harm reduction services, leading to untreated medical conditions, increased risk of infectious diseases, and higher rates of overdose deaths.

Incarceration itself poses health risks, including exposure to violence, inadequate healthcare, and mental health challenges. Formerly incarcerated individuals often struggle to reintegrate into society, facing obstacles such as housing insecurity, unemployment, and lack of access to healthcare.

Moreover, punitive drug policies can undermine public health efforts by discouraging drug users from seeking help and engaging in risky behaviors, such as sharing needles or avoiding overdose prevention measures. This perpetuates a cycle of harm and hinders efforts to address the underlying causes of drug abuse and addiction.

6.4 Racial Disparities and Social Justice

The War on Drugs has been criticized for its disproportionate impact on racial and ethnic minorities, particularly African American and

Latino communities. Racial profiling, discriminatory sentencing practices, and disparities in law enforcement have resulted in higher rates of arrest, conviction, and incarceration for people of color.

The 100:1 sentencing disparity between crack and powder cocaine offenses, for example, disproportionately affected African Americans, who were more likely to be charged with crack-related offenses. This disparity has been widely condemned as discriminatory and unjust, contributing to mass incarceration and racialized policing practices.

The War on Drugs has also contributed to the militarization of police forces and the erosion of civil liberties, particularly in communities of color. Heavy-handed tactics, such as no-knock raids and aggressive policing strategies, have led to increased tensions and distrust between law enforcement and marginalized communities.

6.5 Environmental Impact

The environmental impact of the War on Drugs is often overlooked but significant. Aerial fumigation, used in drug eradication efforts, can lead to deforestation, soil degradation, and contamination of water sources. Chemicals used in drug production, such as methamphetamine labs, pose risks to ecosystems and public health.

The illicit drug trade also contributes to environmental degradation through illegal logging, wildlife trafficking, and habitat destruction in drug-producing regions. These activities have far-reaching ecological consequences, affecting biodiversity, ecosystem services, and environmental sustainability.

Addressing the environmental impact of the War on Drugs requires a comprehensive approach that balances conservation efforts with drug control measures. Sustainable development strategies, alternative livelihoods for affected communities, and environmental regulations can help mitigate the environmental costs of drug production and trafficking.

Chapter 7: Alternatives and Reform in Drug Policy

7.1 Shifts in Public Opinion

Public opinion regarding drug policy has evolved significantly in recent years, reflecting changing attitudes towards drug use, addiction, and criminal justice. Growing recognition of the failures and harms of prohibitionist approaches has led to increased support for alternative drug policies based on public health, harm reduction, and social justice.

Polls and surveys indicate that a majority of Americans now favor decriminalization or legalization of marijuana, reflecting shifting perceptions of cannabis as a less harmful substance than previously believed. Similarly, there is growing support for treatment-focused approaches to drug addiction, emphasizing prevention, education, and rehabilitation over punishment.

7.2 State-Level Reforms

Several U.S. states have enacted significant reforms in drug policy, particularly regarding marijuana legalization and decriminalization. Beginning with California's passage of Proposition 215 in 1996, which legalized medical marijuana, a wave of state-level initiatives has expanded access to cannabis for both medical and recreational use.

As of [insert current year], [number] states and the District of Columbia have legalized recreational marijuana, while [number] states have decriminalized possession of small amounts of cannabis. These reforms reflect a growing acknowledgment of the benefits of regulating and taxing marijuana, reducing law enforcement resources devoted to low-level drug offenses, and addressing racial disparities in drug enforcement.

7.3 International Models of Drug Policy Reform

Several countries have implemented innovative drug policy reforms that depart from traditional prohibitionist approaches. These models offer valuable lessons for addressing the harms of drug abuse and addiction while promoting public health, human rights, and social inclusion.

The Netherlands: Harm Reduction and Cannabis Tolerance

The Netherlands is renowned for its harm reduction approach to drug policy, exemplified by its tolerance of cannabis use in designated coffee shops. The Dutch government prioritizes public health and harm reduction, providing access to clean syringes, opioid substitution therapy, and supervised drug consumption rooms for intravenous drug users.

Portugal: Decriminalization and Public Health

Portugal's decriminalization model, introduced in 2001, treats drug possession for personal use as an administrative rather than criminal offense. Individuals found with small amounts of drugs are referred to a "dissuasion commission" that assesses their needs and recommends treatment, counseling, or fines. The approach emphasizes prevention, treatment, and harm reduction while reducing stigma and criminalization.

Switzerland: Heroin-Assisted Treatment and Harm Reduction

Switzerland's heroin-assisted treatment program provides medically prescribed heroin to individuals with severe addiction who have not responded to other treatments. The program includes comprehensive healthcare, social services, and psychosocial support, leading to improved health outcomes, reduced crime, and social reintegration for participants.

These international models demonstrate that alternative drug policies focused on harm reduction, treatment, and public health can achieve positive outcomes while minimizing the harms associated with punitive approaches.

7.4 Challenges and Barriers to Reform

Despite growing support for drug policy reform, several challenges and barriers persist in implementing alternative approaches. Political resistance, vested interests in the status quo, and ideological opposition to drug liberalization remain significant obstacles to change.

Law enforcement agencies, private prison operators, and other stakeholders with financial incentives tied to drug prohibition often oppose reform efforts that could reduce their influence and funding. The fear of increased drug use, addiction rates, and public safety concerns also deters policymakers from embracing more progressive policies.

Social stigma and misinformation about drug use contribute to public reluctance to support reform initiatives. Debates over the appropriate balance between personal freedom, public health, and public safety continue to shape policy discussions and hinder consensus on effective solutions.

7.5 Opportunities for Reform and Innovation

Despite the challenges, there are promising opportunities for reform and innovation in drug policy. The growing body of evidence supporting public health approaches, harm reduction strategies, and alternatives to incarceration provides a strong foundation for reform advocates.

Community-based initiatives, grassroots movements, and advocacy organizations play a crucial role in raising awareness, mobilizing support, and influencing policy decisions. Collaborative efforts between government agencies, healthcare providers, law enforcement, and civil society can drive meaningful change and promote evidence-based practices.

International cooperation and knowledge-sharing among countries with successful drug policy reforms offer valuable insights and best practices for addressing the global drug problem. Embracing a human rights-based approach, centering the voices of affected communities, and prioritizing harm reduction and social justice are key principles guiding reform efforts.

7.6 The Role of Education and Public Awareness

Education and public awareness campaigns are essential components of drug policy reform, challenging misconceptions, reducing stigma, and promoting evidence-based information. Public engagement, community dialogue, and media literacy efforts can empower individuals to make informed choices about drug use and support harm reduction initiatives.

School-based prevention programs, peer education, and targeted outreach to vulnerable populations are effective strategies for promoting healthy behaviors and reducing drug-related harms. Emphasizing harm reduction principles, such as overdose prevention, safe drug use practices, and access to naloxone, can save lives and prevent unnecessary suffering.

Chapter 8: Human Rights and Drug Policy

8.1 Human Rights Considerations

Drug policy intersects with human rights in significant ways, raising complex ethical and legal questions about individual autonomy, privacy, due process, and access to healthcare. The criminalization of drug use and possession often infringes on fundamental rights, including the right to freedom from discrimination, the right to health, and the right to a fair trial.

Prohibitionist drug policies have led to widespread human rights violations, such as arbitrary arrests, excessive use of force by law enforcement, and harsh sentencing practices. Vulnerable populations, including people who use drugs, ethnic minorities, and marginalized communities, are disproportionately affected by these abuses.

A human rights-based approach to drug policy emphasizes the protection of individual rights, dignity, and autonomy. It prioritizes harm reduction, access to healthcare, and alternatives to incarceration, recognizing that punitive measures often exacerbate social inequalities and violate human rights norms.

8.2 International Human Rights Standards

International human rights law provides a framework for evaluating drug policies and addressing human rights violations in the context of drug control. Treaties such as the Universal Declaration of Human Rights, the International Covenant on Civil and Political Rights, and the International Covenant on Economic, Social and Cultural Rights establish fundamental rights and freedoms that apply to all individuals, including drug users.

Human rights bodies, such as the United Nations Human Rights Council and the Inter-American Commission on Human Rights, monitor compliance with human rights standards and address violations related to drug policies. These bodies have raised concerns about arbitrary detention, torture, and discrimination against drug users and called for reforms to ensure respect for human rights in drug control efforts.

8.3 Human Rights Impact Assessments

Human rights impact assessments (HRIAs) are valuable tools for evaluating the human rights implications of drug policies and interventions. HRIAs analyze the potential impacts of policies on individual rights, identify risks of human rights violations, and recommend measures to mitigate harms and promote human rights compliance.

Incorporating human rights considerations into drug policy development and implementation helps prevent unintended consequences, uphold legal obligations, and protect the rights of vulnerable populations. HRIAs can inform evidence-based decision-making, foster transparency and accountability, and promote participatory approaches that involve affected communities in policy discussions.

8.4 Public Safety and Human Rights

Balancing public safety objectives with respect for human rights is a central challenge in drug policy. While ensuring community safety and crime prevention are legitimate goals, policies that prioritize punitive measures over human rights protections can undermine public trust, exacerbate social tensions, and perpetuate cycles of violence and injustice.

Effective drug policies prioritize harm reduction, prevention, and rehabilitation, recognizing that addressing the root causes of drug abuse and addiction is key to promoting public safety. Community policing, restorative justice approaches, and investment in social services and economic opportunities contribute to safer and more resilient communities.

Human rights principles, such as proportionality, non-discrimination, and accountability, guide efforts to strike a balance between public safety and individual rights. Ensuring access to justice, due process, and accountability mechanisms for human rights violations is essential for building trust in law enforcement and promoting a fair and just society.

8.5 Global Cooperation and Human Rights

International cooperation is essential for promoting human rights in drug policy and addressing transnational challenges related to drug trafficking and organized crime. Collaborative efforts among countries, regional organizations, and civil society actors are key to advancing human rights norms, sharing best practices, and building capacity to implement rights-based approaches.

Global initiatives, such as the United Nations Sustainable Development Goals (SDGs), recognize the interconnectedness of drug policy with broader development, health, and human rights agendas. Goal 3 (Good Health and Well-Being) and Goal 16 (Peace, Justice, and Strong Institutions) underscore the importance of evidence-based drug policies that prioritize public health, human rights, and sustainable development.

Promoting dialogue, knowledge exchange, and mutual support among countries with diverse drug policy experiences fosters a more nuanced and inclusive approach to drug policy reform. Embracing human rights principles as guiding values in international drug control efforts contributes to a more just and humane response to the global drug problem.

Chapter 9: Harm Reduction and Public Health Approaches

9.1 Principles of Harm Reduction

Harm reduction is a pragmatic and compassionate approach to drug policy that prioritizes reducing the negative consequences of drug use rather than solely focusing on abstinence. It is grounded in several key principles:

1. **Human Rights and Dignity:** Recognizing the inherent worth and rights of individuals who use drugs, prioritizing their health, safety, and well-being.
2. **Public Health:** Emphasizing evidence-based interventions that prevent harm, promote health, and reduce the transmission of infectious diseases.
3. **Non-Judgmental Approach:** Avoiding stigmatization, discrimination, and punitive measures, instead fostering open dialogue, empathy, and understanding.
4. **Empowerment:** Engaging drug users as active participants in decision-making, treatment planning, and harm reduction strategies, respecting their autonomy and agency.
5. **Pragmatism:** Acknowledging that abstinence may not be achievable or desirable for everyone, focusing on realistic goals and harm minimization.

9.2 Harm Reduction Interventions

Harm reduction encompasses a range of evidence-based interventions and strategies aimed at reducing the harms associated with drug use. Some common harm reduction interventions include:

- **Needle and Syringe Programs (NSPs):** Providing access to sterile injection equipment, reducing the risk of bloodborne infections such as HIV and hepatitis C among injecting drug users.

- **Opioid Substitution Therapy (OST):** Offering medications like methadone or buprenorphine to treat opioid addiction, reducing cravings, withdrawal symptoms, and illicit drug use.
- **Supervised Injection Facilities (SIFs):** Providing a safe, hygienic environment for drug users to inject drugs under medical supervision, preventing overdoses, and connecting users with healthcare and social services.
- **Naloxone Distribution:** Distributing naloxone, a medication that reverses opioid overdoses, to drug users, their peers, and community members to save lives in case of overdose emergencies.
- **Drug Checking Services:** Offering drug testing services to help users identify the contents and potency of substances, reducing the risk of accidental overdoses and adverse reactions.
- **Education and Counseling:** Providing information, resources, and support to drug users on safer drug use practices, overdose prevention, and accessing healthcare and treatment services.

9.3 Evidence-Based Practices

Harm reduction interventions are grounded in scientific evidence and best practices, informed by research, evaluation, and community input. Evaluating the effectiveness of harm reduction programs involves assessing outcomes such as reduced drug-related harm, improved health outcomes, increased access to services, and changes in drug use behaviors.

Research has consistently shown that harm reduction approaches are effective in reducing the spread of infectious diseases, preventing overdose deaths, improving treatment outcomes, and promoting safer drug use practices. These interventions also contribute to cost savings by reducing healthcare costs, law enforcement expenditures, and social harms associated with drug use.

9.4 Challenges and Opportunities in Harm Reduction

Despite the proven benefits of harm reduction, challenges and barriers persist in implementing these approaches:

- **Stigma and Opposition:** Negative attitudes, misconceptions, and moral objections to drug use and harm reduction can hinder support and funding for these interventions.
- **Legal and Policy Barriers:** Legal restrictions, regulatory challenges, and punitive drug laws can limit the availability and accessibility of harm reduction services.
- **Resource Allocation:** Limited funding, competing priorities, and resource constraints in healthcare systems can impede the scale-up and sustainability of harm reduction programs.
- **Community Engagement:** Building trust, engaging stakeholders, and involving affected communities in planning and implementation are essential for the success of harm reduction initiatives.

Opportunities for advancing harm reduction include:

- **Advocacy and Education:** Raising awareness, challenging stigma, and advocating for policy reform and funding support for harm reduction programs.

- **Collaboration and Partnerships:** Building partnerships across sectors, including healthcare, law enforcement, government agencies, and civil society, to coordinate efforts and leverage resources.
- **Research and Innovation:** Investing in research, data collection, and evaluation to generate evidence, improve program effectiveness, and develop innovative harm reduction interventions.
- **Global Cooperation:** Sharing best practices, lessons learned, and experiences among countries and regions to promote a global culture of harm reduction and public health.

9.5 Integrating Harm Reduction into Drug Policy

Integrating harm reduction principles into drug policy requires a comprehensive and collaborative approach that addresses the complex needs of drug users, communities, and healthcare systems. Key strategies for integrating harm reduction include:

- **Policy Reform:** Reviewing and revising drug laws, regulations, and enforcement practices to prioritize harm reduction, public health, and human rights.
- **Capacity Building:** Strengthening healthcare infrastructure, training healthcare providers, and expanding access to harm reduction services in communities.
- **Community Engagement:** Engaging affected communities, advocating for their needs, and involving them in decision-making and program development.
- **Data Collection and Monitoring:** Establishing systems for data collection, monitoring, and evaluation to track progress, identify gaps, and inform evidence-based decision-making.
- **Collaboration and Coordination:** Building partnerships

among government agencies, civil society organizations, academic institutions, and international partners to coordinate efforts and share resources.

By adopting a harm reduction approach, drug policies can shift from punitive measures to compassionate and effective strategies that prioritize health, safety, and human rights for all individuals affected by drug use.

Chapter 10: Education, Prevention, and Treatment

10.1 Importance of Education and Prevention

Education and prevention are fundamental pillars of effective drug policy, aiming to empower individuals, families, and communities with knowledge, skills, and resources to make informed decisions and prevent drug-related harms. Key aspects of education and prevention include:

- **Public Awareness:** Raising awareness about the risks and consequences of drug use, promoting healthy behaviors, and challenging myths and misconceptions.
- **Youth Education:** Providing age-appropriate education and prevention programs in schools, youth organizations, and community settings to empower young people to make positive choices.
- **Parental Guidance:** Supporting parents and caregivers with information, guidance, and resources to discuss drugs with their children, set boundaries, and promote healthy family environments.
- **Community Engagement:** Engaging communities in prevention efforts, fostering collaboration among stakeholders, and addressing local risk factors and protective factors related to drug use.

10.2 Evidence-Based Prevention Strategies

Evidence-based prevention strategies are grounded in research, data, and best practices, focusing on risk and protective factors that influence drug use behaviors. Some effective prevention strategies include:

- **Life Skills Training:** Teaching interpersonal, communication, problem-solving, and coping skills to enhance resilience and reduce risk factors for drug use among young people.
- **Social Norms Campaigns:** Correcting misperceptions about drug use prevalence and attitudes, promoting positive social norms, and reducing peer pressure to use drugs.
- **Community Programs:** Implementing community-based prevention programs that involve multiple sectors, such as schools, law enforcement, healthcare, and businesses, to address environmental factors contributing to drug use.
- **Media Literacy:** Developing media literacy skills to critically analyze and evaluate media messages about drugs, reduce media influence on drug-related behaviors, and promote responsible media reporting.

10.3 Early Intervention and Treatment

Early intervention and treatment are critical components of drug policy, offering support, counseling, and healthcare services to individuals struggling with drug use disorders. Key aspects of early intervention and treatment include:

- **Screening and Assessment:** Identifying individuals at risk of drug use disorders through screening tools, assessments, and clinical evaluations to determine appropriate interventions.
- **Brief Interventions:** Providing brief counseling, motivational interviewing, and harm reduction strategies to individuals with mild or moderate drug use problems to reduce harm and prevent escalation.
- **Specialized Treatment:** Offering evidence-based treatments, such as cognitive-behavioral therapy, contingency

management, and medication-assisted treatment, tailored to the needs of individuals with severe addiction.

- **Recovery Support Services:** Providing ongoing support, peer counseling, mutual aid groups (e.g., Narcotics Anonymous, SMART Recovery), and relapse prevention strategies to help individuals maintain recovery and improve quality of life.

10.4 Integrating Prevention and Treatment

Integrating prevention and treatment efforts enhances the effectiveness of drug policy by addressing the continuum of care from prevention to recovery. Strategies for integrating prevention and treatment include:

- **Collaborative Approaches:** Fostering collaboration among prevention providers, treatment providers, community organizations, and healthcare systems to coordinate services, share resources, and support seamless transitions for individuals seeking help.
- **Early Identification:** Training frontline professionals, such as educators, healthcare providers, law enforcement officers, and community workers, to recognize signs of drug use, conduct screenings, and refer individuals to appropriate services.
- **Comprehensive Care:** Offering comprehensive care that addresses the complex needs of individuals with drug use disorders, including mental health support, social services, housing assistance, vocational training, and family involvement.
- **Continuum of Services:** Providing a continuum of services, from prevention programs for at-risk populations to intensive treatment for individuals with severe addiction, to ensure a

comprehensive and accessible system of care.

10.5 Challenges and Opportunities in Treatment

Challenges and barriers in treatment include:

- **Stigma and Discrimination:** Overcoming stigma, discrimination, and misconceptions about addiction and treatment to promote acceptance, understanding, and support for individuals seeking help.
- **Access and Equity:** Addressing disparities in access to treatment based on factors such as income, race, ethnicity, geography, and insurance coverage to ensure equitable access to quality care for all.
- **Retention and Engagement:** Improving retention and engagement in treatment by offering personalized, culturally competent, and holistic care that addresses individual needs, preferences, and motivations.
- **Continuity of Care:** Ensuring continuity of care through transitions between different levels of care, settings, and providers to support long-term recovery and prevent relapse.

Opportunities for enhancing treatment include:

- **Evidence-Based Practices:** Implementing evidence-based treatments, protocols, and guidelines based on scientific research and best practices to improve treatment outcomes and quality of care.
- **Innovative Approaches:** Exploring innovative approaches, such as telemedicine, digital health tools, peer support networks, and integrated care models, to expand access, enhance engagement, and support recovery.

- **Community Support:** Mobilizing community support, resources, and partnerships to create supportive environments, reduce barriers to treatment, and promote recovery-oriented systems of care.
- **Policy and Advocacy:** Advocating for policy reforms, funding support, and public investments in addiction treatment, mental health services, and social determinants of health to strengthen the treatment infrastructure and improve outcomes for individuals and communities.

10.6 The Role of Research and Evaluation (continued)

- **Innovation and Technology:** Exploring innovative approaches, technologies, and digital health solutions (e.g., mobile apps, telemedicine, virtual reality) to enhance access, engagement, and outcomes in drug prevention, treatment, and harm reduction.
- **Data Analytics:** Leveraging data analytics, artificial intelligence, and machine learning to analyze patterns, trends, and outcomes in drug use, inform decision-making, and improve the effectiveness of interventions.
- **Evaluating Policy Impact:** Assessing the impact of drug policies, regulations, and interventions on public health, safety, human rights, and social outcomes to inform evidence-based policymaking and advocacy efforts.
- **Longitudinal Studies:** Conducting longitudinal studies and cohort analyses to track changes in drug use patterns, treatment outcomes, and recovery trajectories over time, providing insights into long-term impacts and factors influencing success.
- **Health Economics:** Conducting cost-effectiveness analyses,

economic evaluations, and return on investment studies to assess the economic benefits and value of drug prevention, treatment, and harm reduction interventions, guiding resource allocation and policy priorities.

- **Community-Based Research:** Engaging communities, stakeholders, and affected populations in participatory research, community needs assessments, and program evaluations to ensure relevance, cultural competence, and sustainability of interventions.

10.7 Technology and Innovation in Drug Policy

Technology and innovation play a transformative role in shaping drug policy, enhancing service delivery, and addressing emerging challenges in drug use and addiction. Key areas of technology and innovation in drug policy include:

- **Digital Health Tools:** Utilizing mobile apps, web platforms, and electronic health records to facilitate access to information, education, screening, and support services for individuals with drug use disorders, promoting self-management and engagement in care.

- **Telemedicine and Telehealth:** Expanding access to telemedicine and telehealth services, including virtual counseling, medication management, and remote monitoring, to reach underserved populations, improve continuity of care, and enhance treatment outcomes.

- **Big Data and Analytics:** Harnessing big data analytics, predictive modeling, and data visualization tools to analyze complex datasets, identify trends, patterns, and risk factors in drug use, inform targeted interventions, and evaluate program effectiveness.

- **Artificial Intelligence (AI):** Leveraging AI algorithms, natural language processing, and machine learning techniques to automate processes, personalize interventions, and optimize decision-making in drug prevention, treatment planning, and patient management.
- **Virtual Reality (VR) and Augmented Reality (AR):** Using VR and AR technologies for immersive therapeutic interventions, exposure therapy, skills training, and relapse prevention strategies in addiction treatment, enhancing engagement, motivation, and treatment outcomes.
- **Blockchain Technology:** Exploring blockchain solutions for secure, transparent, and tamper-proof data management, supply chain tracking (e.g., pharmaceuticals, controlled substances), and payment systems in drug policy enforcement, regulatory compliance, and public health surveillance.

10.8 Emerging Issues and Future Directions

As drug policy evolves in response to changing trends, emerging challenges, and technological advancements, several key issues and future directions are worth considering:

- **Polydrug Use and Polysubstance Use:** Addressing the complexities of polydrug use and polysubstance use, including interactions between drugs, co-occurring mental health disorders, and unique treatment needs, through integrated, multidisciplinary approaches.
- **Novel Psychoactive Substances (NPS):** Monitoring and responding to the proliferation of NPS, designer drugs, and synthetic opioids, leveraging rapid detection technologies, forensic analysis, and early warning systems to identify new

substances, assess risks, and inform regulatory measures.

- **Digital Therapeutics:** Exploring the potential of digital therapeutics, gamification, and immersive technologies in delivering evidence-based interventions, behavioral therapies, and cognitive interventions for substance use disorders, enhancing accessibility, engagement, and scalability.

- **Precision Medicine:** Advancing precision medicine approaches, pharmacogenomics, and biomarker research to personalize treatment strategies, predict treatment response, and optimize medication-assisted treatments (e.g., opioid agonists, antagonist medications) based on individual genetic, physiological, and clinical factors.

- **Global Collaboration:** Strengthening international collaboration, information sharing, and capacity-building efforts among countries, regions, and stakeholders to address transnational drug challenges, combat illicit drug trafficking, and promote evidence-based drug policies that prioritize public health, human rights, and social justice.

10.9 Conclusion

In conclusion, education, prevention, treatment, innovation, and research are integral components of comprehensive drug policy approaches. By embracing evidence-based practices, leveraging technology and innovation, and fostering collaboration among stakeholders, policymakers can develop more effective, compassionate, and sustainable solutions to address the complex challenges of drug use and addiction.

Chapter 11: Globalization, International Cooperation, and Cultural Perspectives

11.1 Globalization and Drug Policy

Globalization has profoundly influenced drug policy by shaping patterns of drug production, distribution, consumption, and regulation on a global scale. Key aspects of globalization in drug policy include:

- **Transnational Drug Trade:** The globalization of trade and transportation networks has facilitated the transnational flow of illicit drugs, leading to complex supply chains, organized crime networks, and cross-border challenges in drug enforcement and control.

- **International Drug Treaties:** Global drug control is governed by international treaties such as the Single Convention on Narcotic Drugs (1961), the Convention on Psychotropic Substances (1971), and the United Nations Convention against Illicit Traffic in Narcotic Drugs and Psychotropic Substances (1988), which establish a framework for international cooperation, regulation, and enforcement of drug laws.

- **Cross-Border Collaboration:** International cooperation among law enforcement agencies, customs authorities, and judicial systems is essential for combating transnational drug trafficking, sharing intelligence, extraditing suspects, and prosecuting drug-related crimes across borders.

- **Global Drug Trends:** Globalization has contributed to the spread of drug use trends, cultural influences, and consumption patterns across regions, highlighting the interconnectedness of drug issues and the need for coordinated responses at the international level.

11.2 International Cooperation in Drug Policy

Effective drug policy requires robust international cooperation, coordination, and collaboration among countries, regions, and international organizations. Key aspects of international cooperation in drug policy include:

- **United Nations Office on Drugs and Crime (UNODC):** The UNODC plays a central role in promoting international cooperation, providing technical assistance, capacity-building support, and policy guidance to member states in addressing drug-related challenges.
- **International Drug Control Conventions:** Multilateral agreements and conventions, such as the three UN drug control conventions mentioned earlier, serve as frameworks for harmonizing drug laws, sharing information, and coordinating efforts to prevent drug abuse, trafficking, and diversion.
- **Regional Partnerships:** Regional organizations, such as the European Monitoring Centre for Drugs and Drug Addiction (EMCDDA), the Organization of American States (OAS), and the Association of Southeast Asian Nations (ASEAN), facilitate regional cooperation, data exchange, and policy harmonization in addressing drug issues.
- **Bilateral Agreements:** Bilateral agreements between countries and mutual legal assistance treaties (MLATs) facilitate collaboration in drug enforcement, extradition of suspects, asset forfeiture, and joint operations targeting transnational drug trafficking organizations.

- **Task Forces and Working Groups:** International task forces, working groups, and platforms, such as the International Narcotics Control Board (INCB) and the International Consortium on Drug Policy (ICDP), promote dialogue, information sharing, and best practices exchange among policymakers, experts, and stakeholders.

11.3 Cultural Perspectives on Drug Policy

Cultural perspectives profoundly influence drug policy by shaping attitudes, beliefs, norms, and practices related to drug use, addiction, and treatment. Key aspects of cultural perspectives on drug policy include:

- **Cultural Values:** Cultural values, traditions, and perceptions of drugs vary widely across societies, influencing policies on drug regulation, criminalization, harm reduction, and treatment approaches.
- **Stigma and Discrimination:** Cultural stigma, stereotypes, and discrimination against drug users can impact access to healthcare, social services, and legal protections, shaping policy responses and public attitudes towards drug-related issues.
- **Indigenous and Traditional Practices:** Indigenous cultures often have traditional practices involving psychoactive substances, medicinal plants, and spiritual ceremonies, raising unique considerations in drug policy that respect cultural heritage, autonomy, and rights.
- **Cultural Competence:** Culturally competent approaches in drug policy involve understanding and respecting diverse cultural perspectives, engaging communities, and tailoring interventions to meet the needs, preferences, and values of

diverse populations.

11.4 Challenges and Opportunities in Global Drug Policy

Challenges and opportunities in global drug policy include:

- **Global Drug Trade:** Addressing the complexity and scale of the global drug trade requires coordinated efforts, intelligence sharing, and interagency cooperation at national, regional, and international levels.
- **Policy Harmonization:** Harmonizing drug policies, regulations, and enforcement practices among countries with diverse legal frameworks, cultural contexts, and public health priorities is a challenge but also an opportunity for shared learning, best practices exchange, and mutual support.
- **Human Rights and Public Health:** Balancing human rights principles, public health objectives, and law enforcement priorities in drug policy requires nuanced approaches, dialogue, and collaboration among stakeholders to promote evidence-based, rights-based, and health-centered responses.
- **Innovation and Adaptation:** Harnessing innovation, technology, and data-driven approaches in drug policy can enhance effectiveness, transparency, and accountability while adapting to evolving drug trends, challenges, and opportunities.

11.5 Cultural Sensitivity and Inclusivity

Cultural sensitivity and inclusivity are essential principles in drug policy that promote respect, diversity, and equity in addressing drug-related issues. Strategies for promoting cultural sensitivity and inclusivity in drug policy include:

- **Community Engagement:** Engaging diverse communities, stakeholders, and affected populations in policy development, implementation, and evaluation processes to ensure representation, participation, and ownership of solutions.
- **Cultural Competence Training:** Providing cultural competence training, education, and awareness programs for policymakers, law enforcement officials, healthcare providers, and service providers to enhance understanding, communication, and responsiveness to cultural differences and needs.
- **Language Access:** Ensuring language access, translation services, and culturally appropriate communication materials in drug education, prevention, treatment, and legal proceedings to facilitate access to information and services for non-native speakers and diverse linguistic communities.
- **Cultural Adaptation of Interventions:** Adapting drug prevention, treatment, and harm reduction interventions to align with cultural beliefs, values, practices, and preferences, promoting relevance, effectiveness, and acceptability among diverse populations.

11.6 Ethical Considerations in Global Drug Policy (continued)

- **Respect for Human Rights:** Upholding fundamental human rights, dignity, autonomy, and non-discrimination in drug policies, enforcement practices, and treatment approaches, recognizing the rights of individuals who use drugs and promoting harm reduction, access to healthcare, and due process.
- **Public Health Principles:** Applying public health principles,

evidence-based approaches, and harm reduction strategies in drug policy to prioritize health outcomes, reduce harm, prevent disease transmission, and promote well-being among individuals, communities, and populations affected by drug use.

- **Equity and Social Justice:** Addressing social determinants of health, structural inequalities, and disparities in drug policy to promote equity, fairness, and social justice, including addressing stigma, discrimination, and barriers to access for marginalized and vulnerable populations.

- **Community Empowerment:** Empowering communities, civil society organizations, and grassroots movements in drug policy advocacy, decision-making, and implementation processes to ensure meaningful participation, accountability, and transparency in policy development and service delivery.

- **Evidence-Based Decision-Making:** Using scientific research, data analysis, evaluation findings, and best practices to inform evidence-based decision-making, policy reforms, resource allocation, and programmatic interventions in drug policy.

- **Ethical Oversight:** Establishing ethical oversight mechanisms, accountability frameworks, and human rights monitoring mechanisms in drug policy to prevent abuses, protect vulnerable populations, and uphold ethical standards in law enforcement, healthcare, and treatment settings.

11.7 Impact of Global Drug Policy on Public Health

Global drug policy has significant implications for public health outcomes, healthcare systems, and population well-being. Key aspects of the impact of global drug policy on public health include:

- **Drug-Related Harms:** Drug policies can influence patterns of drug use, availability, purity, potency, and routes of administration, impacting risks of overdose, infectious diseases (e.g., HIV, hepatitis C), mental health disorders, and other drug-related harms among individuals and communities.
- **Access to Healthcare:** Drug policies can affect access to healthcare services, including harm reduction interventions, addiction treatment, mental health support, and primary care, influencing health outcomes, treatment engagement, and continuity of care for individuals with drug use disorders.
- **Health Inequities:** Drug policies can contribute to health inequities, disparities, and barriers to access based on factors such as income, race, ethnicity, gender, sexual orientation, age, disability, and geographic location, highlighting the importance of addressing social determinants of health in drug policy responses.
- **Prevention and Education:** Drug policies can shape prevention efforts, education programs, and public awareness campaigns about drug use risks, harm reduction strategies, overdose prevention, and treatment options, influencing knowledge, attitudes, and behaviors related to drug use and health-seeking behaviors.
- **Health System Resilience:** Drug policies can impact the capacity, resources, and resilience of healthcare systems to respond to drug-related challenges, including addressing substance use disorders, co-occurring health conditions, and public health emergencies (e.g., opioid epidemic, drug-related outbreaks).

11.8 Human Rights and Drug Policy Enforcement

The enforcement of drug policies raises important human rights considerations related to law enforcement practices, criminal justice systems, and individual rights protections. Key aspects of human rights and drug policy enforcement include:

- **Due Process and Legal Protections:** Ensuring due process rights, fair trial standards, legal representation, and access to justice for individuals accused of drug offenses, safeguarding against arbitrary detention, coercion, torture, and violations of privacy rights.

- **Non-Discrimination and Equality:** Promoting non-discrimination, equality, and non-stigmatization in drug policy enforcement, addressing racial profiling, ethnic disparities, gender biases, and other forms of discrimination in policing, prosecution, and sentencing.

- **Alternatives to Incarceration:** Supporting alternatives to incarceration, diversion programs, restorative justice approaches, and community-based sanctions for non-violent drug offenses, emphasizing rehabilitation, reintegration, and social support over punitive measures.

- **Humanitarian and Health-Centered Approaches:** Emphasizing humanitarian, health-centered approaches in drug policy enforcement, prioritizing harm reduction, overdose prevention, access to healthcare, and rights-based interventions for individuals who use drugs, including diversion to treatment programs rather than criminal sanctions.

- **Police Training and Accountability:** Providing training, guidance, and accountability mechanisms for law enforcement officers on human rights, cultural competence, de-escalation techniques, harm reduction principles, and non-coercive approaches in drug-related interactions.

11.9 Global Drug Policy Reform Movements

Global drug policy reform movements advocate for evidence-based, human rights-centered approaches that prioritize public health, harm reduction, social justice, and human rights. Key elements of global drug policy reform movements include:

- **Decriminalization:** Advocating for the decriminalization of drug possession for personal use, shifting from punitive criminal sanctions to public health responses, harm reduction services, and diversion to treatment and support programs.
- **Legalization:** Debating the legalization and regulation of certain drugs, such as cannabis, for medical use, recreational use, or harm reduction purposes, exploring models of legal production, distribution, and consumption that prioritize safety, quality, and public health.
- **Harm Reduction:** Promoting harm reduction as a core principle in drug policy, expanding access to harm reduction interventions (e.g., needle exchange programs, supervised consumption sites, naloxone distribution) to reduce drug-related harms, prevent overdoses, and save lives.
- **Treatment and Support Services:** Advocating for increased funding, resources, and access to evidence-based addiction treatment, mental health services, social support programs, and wraparound services for individuals with drug use disorders, emphasizing recovery-oriented care, peer support, and community integration.
- **Human Rights Protections:** Calling for the protection of human rights, dignity, autonomy, and non-discrimination in drug policy, challenging human rights abuses, systemic

inequalities, and structural barriers that impact vulnerable populations, including people who use drugs, ethnic minorities, and marginalized communities.

11.10 Cultural Diversity and Adaptation in Drug Policy (continued)

- **Cross-Cultural Collaboration:** Fostering cross-cultural collaboration, knowledge exchange, and partnerships among diverse stakeholders, including indigenous communities, immigrant populations, and minority groups, to co-create solutions that are culturally sensitive, inclusive, and effective in addressing drug-related challenges.
- **Cultural Competence Training:** Providing cultural competence training, cultural awareness programs, and diversity education for professionals working in drug policy, law enforcement, healthcare, education, and social services to enhance understanding, respect, and responsiveness to cultural diversity.
- **Cultural Impact Assessment:** Conducting cultural impact assessments, community consultations, and cultural competency audits in drug policy development, implementation, and evaluation processes to identify cultural barriers, disparities, and opportunities for adaptation.
- **Language Access:** Ensuring language access, interpreter services, and multilingual resources in drug education, prevention materials, treatment programs, and legal proceedings to facilitate communication, comprehension, and engagement for linguistically diverse populations.
- **Cultural Safety:** Promoting cultural safety, trust, and rapport in drug policy interactions, service delivery, and

community engagement efforts by creating inclusive, welcoming environments that respect cultural identities, values, and preferences.

- **Ethnic and Indigenous Perspectives:** Incorporating ethnic, indigenous, and traditional knowledge, practices, and perspectives into drug policy discussions, decision-making processes, and program design to honor cultural heritage, resilience, and self-determination.
- **Cultural Sensitivity in Law Enforcement:** Training law enforcement officers on cultural sensitivity, de-escalation techniques, and community policing strategies that prioritize respect, dialogue, and collaboration with diverse communities, reducing tensions, and promoting trust-building efforts.

11.11 Community Engagement and Empowerment

Community engagement and empowerment are essential components of effective drug policy that promote participation, ownership, and accountability among affected populations. Key elements of community engagement and empowerment in drug policy include:

- **Community-Based Approaches:** Adopting community-based approaches in drug policy that involve affected communities, grassroots organizations, civil society groups, and advocacy networks in decision-making, program planning, implementation, and evaluation processes.
- **Community Needs Assessment:** Conducting community needs assessments, asset mapping, and participatory research to identify priorities, strengths, challenges, and resources within communities related to drug use, addiction, prevention, treatment, and harm reduction.

- **Community Mobilization:** Mobilizing communities, building coalitions, and empowering local leaders, activists, and change agents to advocate for policy reforms, funding allocations, and resource investments that address community needs, promote social justice, and reduce drug-related harms.

- **Peer Support and Advocacy:** Fostering peer support networks, mutual aid groups, and peer-led initiatives that provide emotional support, practical guidance, and advocacy opportunities for individuals affected by drug use disorders, promoting solidarity, resilience, and collective action.

- **Community Education and Outreach:** Providing community education, outreach, and awareness campaigns on drug-related risks, harm reduction strategies, treatment options, and legal rights to empower community members with knowledge, skills, and resources to make informed decisions and take action.

- **Capacity Building:** Building community capacity, leadership skills, organizational development, and sustainable infrastructure for community-based initiatives, ensuring continuity, impact, and scalability of community-driven efforts in drug policy.

11.12 Indigenous Perspectives on Drug Policy

Indigenous perspectives on drug policy emphasize cultural sovereignty, self-determination, and holistic approaches that honor indigenous knowledge, traditions, and values. Key elements of indigenous perspectives on drug policy include:

- **Cultural Healing and Wellness:** Emphasizing cultural healing, wellness practices, and traditional medicines as integral components of indigenous approaches to addressing substance use disorders, trauma, intergenerational trauma, and historical trauma.

- **Community-Led Solutions:** Prioritizing community-led solutions, indigenous governance models, and participatory decision-making processes that center the voices, needs, and priorities of indigenous communities in drug policy development, implementation, and evaluation.

- **Cultural Resilience:** Recognizing and promoting cultural resilience, strengths, and protective factors within indigenous communities that contribute to resilience, identity affirmation, and healing in the context of drug-related challenges.

- **Land-Based Healing:** Supporting land-based healing practices, cultural revitalization efforts, and reconnecting indigenous peoples with their traditional lands, languages, ceremonies, and spiritual practices as essential elements of holistic wellness and recovery.

- **Cultural Safety and Trauma-Informed Care:** Implementing culturally safe, trauma-informed approaches in healthcare, social services, and justice systems that respect indigenous worldviews, values, and protocols, addressing historical trauma, systemic injustices, and cultural barriers to care.

- **Indigenous Rights and Self-Governance:** Upholding indigenous rights, self-determination, and treaty rights in drug policy, legal frameworks, and policy dialogues, recognizing indigenous sovereignty, jurisdiction, and authority in addressing drug-related issues within their communities.

11.13 Transnational Drug Policy Challenges

Transnational drug policy challenges require coordinated, collaborative efforts among countries, regions, and international organizations to address complex issues related to drug production, trafficking, consumption, and control. Key transnational drug policy challenges include:

- **Drug Trafficking Routes:** Mapping and disrupting transnational drug trafficking routes, networks, and supply chains that span multiple countries, regions, and continents, leveraging intelligence sharing, interdiction efforts, and international law enforcement cooperation.

- **Border Control and Customs Cooperation:** Strengthening border control measures, customs cooperation, and border security initiatives to detect, intercept, and prevent illicit drug shipments, smuggling activities, and cross-border criminal enterprises.

- **Money Laundering and Financial Crimes:** Combating money laundering, financial crimes, and illicit financial flows associated with drug trafficking through international cooperation, regulatory frameworks, and financial intelligence sharing mechanisms.

- **International Drug Demand Reduction:** Promoting international collaboration on drug demand reduction strategies, prevention programs, treatment services, and harm reduction interventions to address global patterns of drug use, addiction, and public health consequences.

- **Cross-Border Law Enforcement Operations:** Conducting joint law enforcement operations, task forces, and intelligence sharing initiatives among countries and regional organizations to target transnational drug trafficking organizations, disrupt criminal networks, and dismantle illicit drug markets.

- **Diplomatic Engagement and Policy Coordination:** Engaging in diplomatic dialogue, policy coordination, and multilateral agreements among countries, regions, and international bodies (e.g., United Nations, Interpol, World Health Organization) to align drug policies, regulatory frameworks, and enforcement priorities with global public health, human rights, and development goals.

11.14 Global Drug Policy Reform Initiatives (continued)

- **Decriminalization:** Advocating for the decriminalization of drug possession for personal use, shifting from punitive criminal sanctions to public health responses, harm reduction services, and diversion to treatment and support programs.
- **Legalization:** Debating the legalization and regulation of certain drugs, such as cannabis, for medical use, recreational use, or harm reduction purposes, exploring models of legal production, distribution, and consumption that prioritize safety, quality, and public health.
- **Harm Reduction:** Promoting harm reduction as a core principle in drug policy, expanding access to harm reduction interventions (e.g., needle exchange programs, supervised consumption sites, naloxone distribution) to reduce drug-related harms, prevent overdoses, and save lives.
- **Treatment and Support Services:** Advocating for increased funding, resources, and access to evidence-based addiction treatment, mental health services, social support programs, and wraparound services for individuals with drug use disorders, emphasizing recovery-oriented care, peer support,

and community integration.

- **Human Rights Protections:** Calling for the protection of human rights, dignity, autonomy, and non-discrimination in drug policy, challenging human rights abuses, systemic inequalities, and structural barriers that impact vulnerable populations, including people who use drugs, ethnic minorities, and marginalized communities.

11.15 International Cooperation in Drug Policy

International cooperation is essential in addressing transnational drug challenges, promoting shared responsibility, and fostering collaboration among countries, regions, and international organizations. Key elements of international cooperation in drug policy include:

- **United Nations Conventions:** Implementing and adhering to international drug control conventions, treaties, and agreements that provide frameworks for cooperation, regulation, and enforcement of drug laws at the global level.
- **Bilateral and Multilateral Agreements:** Establishing bilateral and multilateral agreements, partnerships, and initiatives among countries, regional organizations, and international bodies to strengthen coordination, intelligence sharing, and joint actions in combating drug trafficking, money laundering, and organized crime.
- **Global Task Forces:** Supporting global task forces, working groups, and platforms, such as the International Narcotics Control Board (INCB), the Global Drug Policy Observatory (GDPO), and the United Nations Office on Drugs and Crime (UNODC), that facilitate information exchange, policy analysis, and capacity-building efforts in drug policy.

- **Interagency Collaboration:** Promoting interagency collaboration among law enforcement agencies, customs authorities, public health agencies, diplomatic missions, and civil society organizations to address multidimensional aspects of drug-related challenges, including supply reduction, demand reduction, and harm reduction strategies.
- **International Funding and Assistance:** Providing international funding, technical assistance, and capacity-building support to developing countries, vulnerable regions, and affected communities to strengthen drug prevention, treatment, and law enforcement capabilities, enhance regulatory frameworks, and promote sustainable development goals.
- **Diplomatic Engagement:** Engaging in diplomatic dialogue, policy coordination, and diplomatic negotiations at bilateral, regional, and international forums to address cross-border drug issues, policy harmonization, and mutual cooperation in drug control efforts.

11.16 Emerging Trends in Drug Policy

Emerging trends in drug policy reflect evolving challenges, innovations, and responses to changing patterns of drug use, trafficking, and regulation. Key emerging trends in drug policy include:

- **New Psychoactive Substances (NPS):** Monitoring and responding to the proliferation of new psychoactive substances, synthetic drugs, and designer substances that pose challenges in regulation, detection, and risk assessment, requiring agile regulatory frameworks, forensic capabilities, and public health responses.
- **Cannabis Legalization:** The growing trend towards cannabis

legalization and regulation for medical and recreational use in various countries and jurisdictions, raising questions about market regulation, public health impacts, youth access, and international drug treaty compliance.

- **Opioid Epidemic Response:** Addressing the opioid epidemic and opioid crisis through comprehensive strategies that combine prevention, treatment expansion, harm reduction interventions (e.g., naloxone distribution, syringe exchange programs), and enforcement measures to reduce opioid-related overdoses, deaths, and addiction rates.

- **Digital Drug Markets:** Responding to the emergence of digital drug markets, online drug sales, and darknet platforms that facilitate illicit drug transactions, posing challenges in law enforcement, regulatory control, and international cooperation in combating cybercrime and illicit online activities.

- **Medicalization of Drug Policy:** The shift towards medicalization, harm reduction, and public health approaches in drug policy that prioritize evidence-based interventions, treatment access, and harm reduction services for individuals with substance use disorders, emphasizing health outcomes, human rights, and dignity.

- **Psychedelic Research and Therapies:** The resurgence of interest in psychedelic research, psychedelic-assisted therapies, and the therapeutic potential of psychedelic substances (e.g., psilocybin, MDMA) in mental health treatment, addiction recovery, and trauma healing, leading to discussions about regulatory frameworks, research ethics, and clinical applications.

- **Drug Policy Innovation:** Exploring innovative policy

approaches, pilot programs, and experimental models in drug policy, such as drug checking services, safe consumption spaces, alternative sentencing programs, and community diversion initiatives, to test new strategies, evaluate outcomes, and inform evidence-based practices.

11.7 Case Study: The Philippines and Duterte's Drug War

Overview of President Duterte's Anti-Drug Campaign

President Rodrigo Duterte's anti-drug campaign in the Philippines has been characterized by aggressive tactics, including extrajudicial killings, crackdowns on drug suspects, and a "war on drugs" rhetoric. The campaign, launched in 2016, aimed to eradicate drug-related crime and addiction through a combination of law enforcement measures and harsh penalties.

Human Rights Violations and International Response

The anti-drug campaign has faced widespread criticism for human rights violations, including thousands of extrajudicial killings of suspected drug offenders, arbitrary arrests, and lack of due process. International human rights organizations, such as Human Rights Watch and Amnesty International, have condemned these violations and called for accountability and justice.

Impact on Filipino Society and Potential for Policy Change

The impact of Duterte's drug war on Filipino society has been significant, leading to increased fear, division, and mistrust within communities. The campaign's focus on punitive measures has raised concerns about its effectiveness in addressing root causes of drug use, promoting rehabilitation, and respecting human rights. There is potential for policy change towards a more holistic approach that prioritizes public health, harm reduction, and evidence-based interventions.

11.8 The Role of Social Movements and Advocacy

Analysis of Social Movements Advocating for Drug Policy Reform

Social movements advocating for drug policy reform play a crucial role in challenging punitive approaches, promoting human rights, and advocating for evidence-based solutions. These movements often include diverse stakeholders, such as affected communities, healthcare professionals, academics, legal experts, and civil society organizations, united in their call for more humane and effective drug policies.

Role of Advocacy Organizations and Community Groups

Advocacy organizations and community groups play a vital role in driving policy change, raising awareness, mobilizing public support, and holding policymakers accountable. They engage in various advocacy strategies, such as lobbying, public campaigns, media outreach, legal challenges, and grassroots organizing, to influence drug policy agendas and promote social justice.

Case Studies of Successful Advocacy Efforts

Several case studies illustrate successful advocacy efforts in drug policy reform. For example, the decriminalization of drug possession for personal use in Portugal, coupled with investments in harm reduction and treatment services, has led to positive outcomes in reducing drug-related harms and promoting public health. Similarly, the expansion of harm reduction programs and overdose prevention initiatives in Canada and Australia showcases the impact of advocacy in shaping progressive drug policies.

Chapter 12: The Future of the War on Drugs

12.1 Emerging Drug Trends and Threats

- **Analysis of New and Emerging Drugs:** Investigating the rise of new and potent substances such as synthetic opioids, designer drugs, and novel psychoactive substances (NPS), their chemical compositions, effects, risks, and challenges they pose to public health and law enforcement.

- **Impact of Changing Drug Use Patterns:** Assessing the evolving patterns of drug use, consumption methods, market trends, and user demographics, and their implications for drug policy formulation, enforcement strategies, and harm reduction interventions.

- **Strategies for Addressing Emerging Drug Threats:** Proposing innovative strategies, surveillance systems, early warning mechanisms, and collaborative approaches among policymakers, law enforcement agencies, healthcare providers, and community organizations to address emerging drug threats effectively.

12.2 Technological Innovations in Drug Enforcement

- **Overview of Technological Advancements:** Examining advancements such as big data analytics, artificial intelligence (AI), machine learning, block chain technology, and forensic tools in drug enforcement efforts, including drug detection, supply chain tracking, financial investigations, and predictive modeling.

- **Potential Benefits and Risks:** Analyzing the potential

benefits, risks, ethical considerations, and unintended consequences of adopting new technologies in drug enforcement, including issues related to privacy, data security, algorithm biases, and civil liberties.

- **Future Trends and Implications:** Forecasting future trends in technological innovation within drug enforcement, exploring potential scenarios, policy implications, and regulatory frameworks needed to ensure responsible and effective use of technology in combating drug-related crimes.

12.3 Global Perspectives on Drug Policy

- **Comparative Analysis of Drug Policies:** Conducting a comparative analysis of drug policies across different countries, regions, and cultural contexts, examining variations in approaches to drug regulation, legalization, decriminalization, harm reduction, and public health strategies.
- **Impact of Globalization:** Assessing the impact of globalization, international trade, digital economies, and cross-border flows on drug trafficking, supply chains, enforcement challenges, and policy harmonization efforts at the global level.
- **Role of International Cooperation:** Highlighting the role of international cooperation, diplomatic engagement, multilateral agreements, and collaborative initiatives in shaping future drug policies, promoting shared responsibility, and addressing transnational drug challenges effectively.

12.4 Vision for a Post-Prohibition World

- **Analysis of Post-Prohibition Approaches:** Exploring the feasibility, benefits, risks, and implications of transitioning towards a post-prohibition approach to drug policy, including models of regulated legalization, harm reduction-focused strategies, and alternative frameworks for drug control.

- **Economic, Social, and Public Health Implications:** Evaluating the potential economic impacts, social justice outcomes, public health benefits, and law enforcement considerations of ending prohibition, shifting towards regulation, and redirecting resources towards prevention, treatment, and harm reduction.
- **Roadmap for Transitioning:** Developing a roadmap, policy guidelines, and implementation strategies for transitioning to a post-prohibition world, including stakeholder engagement, legislative reforms, regulatory frameworks, and international coordination efforts.

12.5 Policy Innovations and Best Practices

- **Overview of Innovative Policy Approaches:** Reviewing innovative policy models, pilot programs, and best practices in drug policy from around the world, including successful case studies of policy innovations in prevention, treatment, harm reduction, and law enforcement.
- **Case Studies of Successful Policy Innovations:** Examining case studies of successful policy innovations, including examples of regulatory frameworks, diversion programs, community-based initiatives, and evidence-based interventions that have demonstrated positive outcomes in reducing drug-related harms and improving public health.
- **Recommendations for Implementation:** Providing

recommendations for implementing best practices, scaling up successful interventions, overcoming barriers to policy innovation, and fostering a culture of learning, adaptation, and continuous improvement in drug policy systems.

12.6 Future Directions for Drug Treatment and Harm Reduction

- **Emerging Trends in Addiction Treatment:** Examining emerging trends and innovations in addiction treatment, including evidence-based practices, pharmacological therapies, behavioral interventions, digital health tools, and integrated care models that prioritize holistic approaches, patient-centered care, and long-term recovery outcomes.
- **Role of New Therapies and Technologies:** Assessing the role of new therapies, medications, and technologies in addiction treatment and harm reduction, such as medication-assisted treatment (MAT), telehealth services, mobile applications, virtual reality interventions, and personalized medicine approaches tailored to individual needs and preferences.
- **Policy Implications of Advances:** Discussing the policy implications of advances in addiction treatment and harm reduction, including regulatory frameworks, reimbursement policies, workforce training, quality standards, and access barriers to evidence-based care for individuals with substance use disorders.

12.7 The Role of Education and Public Awareness

- **Importance of Education:** Highlighting the importance of education, prevention, and public awareness campaigns in shaping attitudes, behaviors, and perceptions related to drug use, addiction, treatment, recovery, and harm reduction strategies, targeting diverse audiences, including youth, families, communities, and policymakers.

- **Strategies for Effective Public Education:** Identifying strategies for designing effective public education campaigns, including messaging strategies, media outreach, digital platforms, peer education programs, school-based initiatives, and community engagement efforts that promote accurate information, destigmatize substance use disorders, and encourage help-seeking behaviors.

- **Case Studies of Successful Initiatives:** Showcasing case studies of successful education and awareness initiatives from different regions, highlighting key lessons learned, best practices, evaluation methods, and impact assessments in changing knowledge, attitudes, and behaviors related to drug use and addiction.

12.8 Building a More Just and Effective Drug Policy

- **Key Principles for Just Policy:** Proposing key principles and guiding values for a more just and effective drug policy, including human rights protections, harm reduction approaches, evidence-based practices, health-centered strategies, equity considerations, community engagement, and social justice outcomes.

- **Role of Stakeholders:** Discussing the role of diverse stakeholders, including government agencies, law enforcement, healthcare providers, advocacy organizations, civil society groups, academia, industry partners, and affected communities, in driving policy change, fostering collaboration, and promoting accountability in drug policy decision-making processes.

- **Vision for the Future:** Articulating a vision for the future of drug policy and the War on Drugs that prioritizes public health, human rights, social justice, and community well-being, envisioning a shift towards prevention, treatment, harm reduction, and evidence-based interventions as central pillars of drug policy frameworks.

Chapter 13: Conclusion and Recommendations

13.1 Summary of Key Findings

This section will provide a detailed recap of the major findings from each chapter, synthesizing key insights and conclusions drawn from our comprehensive exploration of drug policy. It will highlight significant trends, challenges, opportunities, and lessons learned throughout the book, offering readers a clear understanding of the complex dynamics and evolving landscape of drug policy.

13.2 Policy Recommendations

In-depth policy recommendations will be provided based on the thorough analysis presented in the book. These recommendations will encompass a wide range of areas within drug policy, including:

- **Prevention:** Strategies for early intervention, youth education programs, community-based prevention initiatives, and public health campaigns targeting substance use disorders.
- **Treatment:** Recommendations for expanding access to evidence-based addiction treatment, integrating mental health services, promoting recovery-oriented care, and addressing gaps in treatment infrastructure.
- **Harm Reduction:** Policies to support harm reduction interventions, such as needle exchange programs, supervised consumption sites, naloxone distribution, and drug checking services, emphasizing public health approaches and reducing harm associated with drug use.
- **Law Enforcement:** Guidelines for shifting law enforcement

priorities towards community policing, diversion programs, alternative sentencing, restorative justice, and reducing incarceration rates for non-violent drug offenses.

- **International Cooperation:** Strategies for enhancing international cooperation, information sharing, capacity-building efforts, and diplomatic engagement to address transnational drug challenges and promote global public health goals.

- **Community Engagement:** Recommendations for empowering communities, fostering collaboration with affected populations, promoting peer support networks, and involving community-based organizations in policy decision-making processes.

13.3 The Path Forward

This section will outline concrete steps needed to move towards a more effective, equitable, and just approach to drug policy. It will address the role of various stakeholders, including:

- **Government Entities:** Advocating for evidence-based policies, resource allocation for prevention and treatment programs, regulatory reforms, and legislative initiatives that prioritize public health and human rights.

- **Healthcare Providers:** Encouraging integration of addiction treatment into primary care, training healthcare professionals in addiction medicine, reducing stigma in healthcare settings, and expanding telehealth services for remote access to treatment.

- **Law Enforcement Agencies:** Promoting diversion programs, crisis intervention training, harm reduction collaboration, community policing models, and decriminalization of low-level drug offenses.

- **Advocacy Groups:** Supporting advocacy efforts for policy reform, grassroots campaigns, public education initiatives, coalition building, and mobilizing public support for evidence-based drug policies.
- **Community Organizations:** Empowering communities to develop tailored solutions, providing social support services, promoting harm reduction practices, and engaging in policy advocacy at the local level.

13.4 Final Reflections

This section will offer deeper reflections on the historical context, policy failures, unintended consequences, and societal impacts of the War on Drugs. It will underscore the need for transformative change, systemic reforms, and addressing structural inequalities within drug policy frameworks. Reflections will also include insights from affected individuals, families, and communities impacted by punitive drug policies.

13.5 Call to Action

The call to action will be robust, encouraging readers to actively engage in drug policy reform efforts. It will provide:

- **Encouragement:** Motivating individuals to advocate for change, share personal stories, challenge stigma, and promote empathy and understanding towards individuals affected by substance use disorders.
- **Resources:** Offering a comprehensive list of resources, including research studies, policy briefs, toolkits, advocacy guides, online platforms, and support networks for individuals interested in drug policy reform.

- **Organizations:** Highlighting key organizations, NGOs, advocacy groups, grassroots movements, and campaigns focused on drug policy reform, human rights, harm reduction, and public health advocacy.
- **Action Steps:** Suggesting specific action steps, such as contacting elected representatives, participating in advocacy campaigns, attending community meetings, supporting harm reduction services, and engaging in public education efforts.

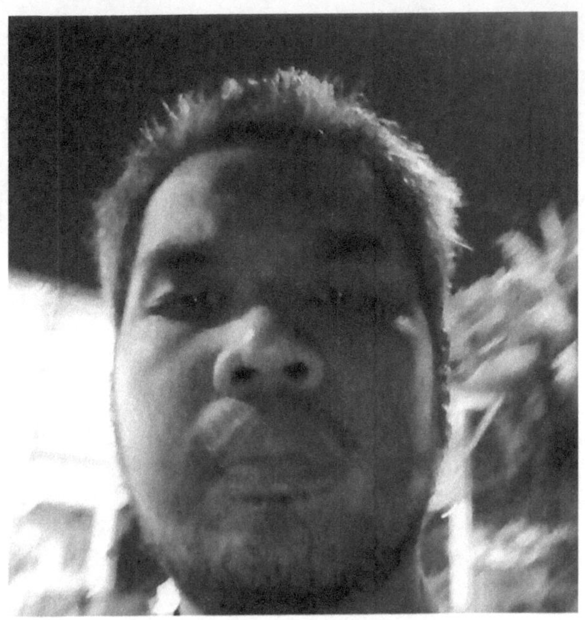

About the Author

Arief Muinnudin was born in Malaysia in 1987, where he discovered his passion for writing at a young age. Growing up surrounded by the diverse cultures and vibrant landscapes of Malaysia, Arief developed a deep appreciation for storytelling and the power of words to connect people from different backgrounds.

From his early years, Arief was drawn to literature and the art of crafting narratives that captivate and inspire readers. He immersed himself in a wide range of genres, from fiction to non-fiction, exploring various themes and styles to hone his writing skills.

As Arief's love for writing blossomed, so did his ambition to share meaningful stories with the world. He embarked on a journey to become a published author, dedicating countless hours to researching, writing, and refining his manuscripts.

With each book he wrote, Arief aimed to engage readers on a profound level, sparking discussions, provoking thought, and leaving a lasting impact on their lives. His commitment to creating compelling and insightful content earned him recognition as a talented writer with a unique voice and perspective.

Arief's passion for literature continues to drive him forward, inspiring him to explore new ideas, tackle challenging topics, and connect with readers on a deeper level through the power of storytelling.

Read more at https://ariefebook.etsy.com.